A QUICK GUIDE TO FOOD SAFETY

Robert L. Goodman

Silvercat Publications
San Diego, California

363.192

1992

Every effort has been made to assure the accuracy of the information presented in this book. However, nothing in this book should be construed as medical advice or used in place of medical consultation.

First Printing, November, 1991   10 9 8 7 6 5 4 3 2 1

Publisher's Cataloging in Publication
(Prepared by Quality Books Inc.)

Goodman, Robert L.
    A quick guide to food safety / Robert L. Goodman
    p. cm.
    Includes bibliographical references.
    ISBN 0-9624945-3-4

    1. Food contamination--Handbooks, manuals, etc. 2. Food additives--Handbooks, manuals, etc. 3. Food adulteration and inspection--Handbooks, manuals, etc. I. Title

TX533   363.192
Library of Congress Catalog Card Number 91-67069

Printed in the United States of America

Table of Contents

Introduction
Food Safety

How safe is the food we eat? Consumers everywhere are beginning to ask questions about chemicals, bacteria, and other substances in their food. Survey after survey reports that food safety has become one of the dominant grocery issues of the 1990s. Consumers have become increasingly worried about the potential health hazards found on their plates and increasingly skeptical about the ability or willingness of government or industry to watch out for the public's health. Statistics give little assurance. Even though no one knows exactly how diet causes cancer, some authorities have estimated that as many cancers are caused each year by diet as are caused by tobacco. The average citizen is often perplexed by chemicals intentionally added to food; by residues of pesticides, hormones, antibiotics, and other chemicals; by naturally occurring microbiological contaminants; by contamination of food by manmade, industrial chemicals; and by so many other potential compromises of the food system.

The problem of food safety is nothing new. Our remote ancestors certainly learned valuable if painful lessons about eating things like oleander or rhubarb leaves, rancid meat, and stagnant water. We have benefited from their collective mistakes. Thanks to their early misfortunes, we have evolved very effective internal immune and detoxifying systems which allow us to resist the effects of many occasional misjudgments.

During the last fifty years, chemistry and technology have dramatically changed the agriculture and food industries. New research has promised new solutions to old and new problems. New techniques, new procedures, new chemicals, and new machines have been developed to tackle the challenges of production, control, efficiency, and distribution. New strains of crops have been designed to combat specific problems or to increase yields.

3

New knowledge about chemical and biological processes has given us new ways to attack traditional problems. And now, as the twenty-first century approaches, the test tube has emerged as the next frontier of applied knowledge.

Substantial progress has been made toward eliminating many traditional safety problems. But new problems continue to surface. Ironically, many of these new problems are caused by the very technology we have used to make our lives better. We develop chemicals and drugs for agricultural and veterinary purposes and find their residues in the foods we eat. Meanwhile, the pests and microorganisms they are supposed to eradicate evolve into new, resistant forms that require more and stronger controls. We add chemicals to foods in the factory and discover that they remain in the food on the plate. We develop new forms of packaging only to find that some of the chemicals used in the packages become part of our food. We process food in the name of convenience even though the extra handling during processing makes bacterial and other forms of contamination more likely. Meanwhile, we centralize food production and distribution into fewer and fewer hands and find that a single accident can now affect far greater numbers of people. So many promising solutions end up creating new challenges of their own.

We are rapidly becoming aware that the food system does not exist outside of the larger world. Everything is related to everything else. Agricultural and industrial chemicals—mercury, PCB's, solvents, heavy metals, etc.—contaminate ground water and fishing areas. The national and international distribution of food places heavy demands on the transportation and fuel systems, adds to air pollution, and possibly contributes to changes in the climate. An agriculture industry which relies heavily on fertilizers and pesticides becomes increasingly committed to the use of still more chemicals, seemingly in disregard of their environmental and human impacts. Meanwhile, existing agricultural lands become lost to development, topsoil erosion, and nutrient depletion, while new agricultural and grazing lands are carved out of rain forests and other previously virgin areas. These are largely technological phenomena that can only be addressed by the application of more technology. Our problems no longer seem solvable by individuals, and the world seems to become so much more complex and beyond our control.

Yet, things are not always as they seem. Individual consumers still have the ability to make a difference. But consumers must exercise this power. It is not enough to sit back, expecting the food industry or the government to watch out for our best interests. If consumers do not act, industry and government will certainly make decisions for us. But then we will have no right to complain when we discover that we do not share their ideas about what our bests interests really are.

Consumers must take initiative if they want to influence the direction of progress or broaden their control over the food on their plates. This book was designed to help consumers make these decisions. It presents the basic facts as impartially as possible so that consumers can make up their own minds. It does not attempt to take sides, but it does advocate, sometimes passionately, the recommendations which appear in its pages. It does not attempt to cast blame or to question the motives of the food industry or its critics. Rather, it accepts that each side has a legitimate perspective, and it attempts to be fair in treating the basic issues of food safety. What matters, after all, is information, not reproach.

Chapter 1
Food Additives

What are food additives? In simple terms, they are any substances which have been added to food, whether accidentally or intentionally. Additives have been used for centuries. People were using ingredients like salt, sugar, spices, and yeast long before the first recipe was written. Even today, these types of substances still make up the bulk (in weight) of all food additives.

During the last two or three decades, however, a host of powerful chemical additives has been developed. Food additives have become big business. In excess of 3,000 different chemicals are now *intentionally* used in processed foods, and industry experts predict that the additives market will double in size during the next decade. The average American eats about 150 pounds of additives each year. Most of these are sugar and salt. But almost 15 pounds are various other chemicals, many of which have been created in the test tube.

The growing use of intentional additives has been paralleled by an equally remarkable increase in the use of other chemicals throughout the food system. Some of these chemicals have been used to boost crop yields or meat production. Others have been used to control the pests and organisms which threaten the food supply. Still others have been used to improve the transportation, storage, and packaging of foods. An increasingly complex food system has made intensive use of technology and chemicals to put foods in the hands and mouths of consumers. Some of these non-food chemicals become the *incidental* additives discussed in Chapter 2.

Collectively, these additives have contributed to a revolution in food technology. Over half the food in grocery stores has appeared within the last ten years, and food technology experts predict that within a decade almost eighty percent of grocery items will be less than ten years old. In 1990 alone, as many as 12,000 new food items were placed on grocery-store shelves. More than half of the typical American diet today consists of processed, packaged, or otherwise engineered foods containing significant amounts of food additives.

The food system cannot be separated from its social and economic context. The number and amount of additives in food has continued to increase because the food industry has willingly responded to new technologies and changing consumer demands. Continuing social and technological change is likely to stimulate even more convenience foods and additives in the future. As long as a society of consumers continues to demand modern and convenient foods, the processed food industry will continue to thrive. And as it does, the number and amount of food additives we consume will inevitably increase.

The Advantages and Disadvantages of Additives

Additives are used because they offer benefits to both consumer and industry. The most obvious benefit is convenience. Additives make the processing, preparing, and cooking of food faster, simpler, and more predictable. Additives make shopping easier, too, by allowing consumers to shop less often and to choose from a greater variety of foods. There are other benefits as well. Additives guard against food spoilage, ensuring an adequate supply of food throughout the country. Along with refrigeration, they help protect consumers from serious, food-related diseases like hepatitis, tuberculosis, trichinosis, botulism, and salmonella. Without additives, many foods would be impossible to manufacture. Some additives make processing possible, while others restore some of the vitamins and nutrients that processing destroys. Finally, additives mean lower production costs, reduced wastes, and greater profits for the food industry and occasionally lower prices for the consumer.

To enjoy all these benefits, however, consumers must pay certain hidden costs. Not all additives are necessary or useful. Some can be harmful. Others are poisons. A number of additives can cause allergic reactions, cancer, birth defects, genetic mutations, heart and organ disease, spontaneous abortions, brain damage, nervousness, learning disorders, behavior problems, tooth decay, and other health problems.

Additives too often are used for "cosmetic" purposes—to improve the way food looks, smells, feels, or tastes. In many refined and "designer" foods, chemicals with no food value are used to replace more expensive but nutritious natural ingredients. Despite industry claims to the contrary, processed foods often cost more than the same foods cooked from scratch. At the same time, additives dilute quality—processed food is never the same as the "real thing." Finally, additives are commonly used in those highly processed, heavily advertised foods which contain undesirable amounts of sugar, salt, and fat. Many of the health problems associated with additives may well be caused, not by the chemicals alone, but also by the commercially successful yet nutritionally deficient foods in which they are used.

Are Additives Safe?

The federal government has attempted to ensure the safe use of additives in food since the passage of the Pure Food and Drug Act of 1906. This federal commitment to safety has been placed primarily in the hands of the Food and Drug Administration (FDA) and, to a lesser extent, the Department of Agriculture (USDA), the Environmental Protection Agency (EPA), and the National Marine Fisheries Service. State and local agencies have also attempted to ensure that only safe chemicals are used in food.

The challenges facing these overworked and understaffed agencies are considerable. Natural and synthetic additives are chemicals which can have direct effects of their own. They can also act like drugs to change the way the body works. Many of these substances have only recently been introduced into the human diet, so the long-term effects of consumption are unknown. Some additives are certainly safe and useful. Others may be safe only some of the time or only for some people. Even some "safe" additives may interact with other chemicals to produce surprising and unpredictable side-effects. Still others, including a number of natural additives, raise unanswered and perhaps unanswerable questions about such health problems as cancer, birth defects, genetic mutations, behavioral changes, food sensitivities, and allergic reactions.

Most additives have been tested for their potential to cause some of these conditions. But testing can never tell if an additive is harmless. A thousand tests cannot prove the safety of an additive, because there can be no assurance that the thousand-and-first test will not reveal a potential hazard. Testing laboratories attempt to prove that a given additive is harmful by asking if a specific amount...of a specific additive (or combination of additives)... causes specific kinds of "statistically significant" damage or change... to specific parts of the body...under specific conditions...within a specific period of time. If the laboratory can determine how the chemical is processed, or *metabolized*, by the body, so much the better. But claims that an additive is safe are often based on a failure to find evidence that it is harmful. And it may take years for evidence sufficient to call an additive into question to be accumulated.

Responsibility for the actual testing rests with the manufacturer, who must evaluate each potentially new additive for its probable safety. (The manufacturer does not need to prove that the additive is necessary, however.) Normally, the testing itself is done by independent laboratories under commission of the manufacturer. Test results are then sent to the FDA, which evaluates the data and determines whether or not the additive may be used in food and what, if any, restrictions will be applied.

Testing standards have become far more rigorous as our knowledge of the subtle and long range effects of additives has increased. Unfortunately, even the most rigorous tests still leave many questions unanswered. Legally, these tests may only be performed on animals, but animals and humans display vastly different reactions, sensitivities, and rates of absorption, metabolism, and toxicity. The resulting "proof by analogy" may or may not reflect the true effects of a given chemical on humans.

Moreover, proper testing is both expensive and time-consuming. Ideally, tests should span multiple generations of animals to determine the long-term effects of normal doses of an additive or a combination of additives. But the manufacturers who pay for the tests are frequently impatient for results. Testing correctly assumes that too much of anything can be harmful. Accordingly, laboratories seek to identify "threshold levels" which define how much of a specific chemical is too much. But critics point out, also correctly, that the idea of a threshold may only be wishful thinking.

At least for some substances, a safe level of consumption may not exist.

Even if the laboratories could overcome these problems, testing would still be inconclusive. Proper, scientific, and acceptable testing can only be performed under clinical conditions which are far removed from the realities of Main Street. Strict controls must be imposed within the laboratory in order to prevent distortions caused by elements not being tested. Thus, extremely healthy animals are kept in sanitary, almost perfect conditions and fed wholesome, controlled diets in order to isolate the effects of everything except the tested chemical. To obtain unambiguous measurements, laboratories often administer these substances in concentrations, dosages, or frequencies which are totally untypical of a normal diet. If the additive "passes" the test, it is then allowed to be used in an imperfect world where people in varying states of health breathe unfiltered air, drink impure water, eat uncontrolled amounts of nutritionally diverse foods, and otherwise expose themselves to influences which could not be permitted in the laboratory. Finally, testing only examines an additive's safety. The laboratory seldom asks whether an additive is nutritionally sound, worthwhile, or necessary.

Some additives are not even tested. The 1958 Food Additives Amendment to the Food, Drug, and Cosmetic Act of 1938 exempted certain substances from testing. These included additives which had been "prior sanctioned" and those which seemed from experience to be safe. This latter category, known as "Generally Recognized as Safe" (GRAS), includes many of the currently most widely used additives as well as a number of "common food ingredients" like salt, pepper, vinegar, baking powder, and MSG. These substances may be used without any limit except for "good manufacturing practices."

No one really knows how many additives are GRAS, because manufacturers themselves can add chemicals to the GRAS list following the completion of tests which the manufacturer feels demonstrate the safety of the additive. Only when the additive is used in food can the FDA declare that the additive needs to be tested further or restricted in some manner. The GRAS classification does not guarantee the safety of an additive. Several formerly GRAS additives, including cyclamates, saccharin, saffrole (a natural flavoring agent extracted from sassafras), brominated vegetable oil, and many artificial colors have been found dangerous and either removed from the GRAS list or banned outright after years of unrestricted use.

The FDA itself admits that "there is no way in which absolute safety can be guaranteed." Too many potential problems exist. Any substance can be harmful when abused. Chemicals which are safe by themselves may be converted to dangerous substances when they are exposed to other chemicals or to digestive enzymes. Other chemicals may produce dangerous by-products when they are metabolized by the body. Substances which are safe for the vast majority of the population may be harmful to sensitive or allergic individuals. Levels of consumption which are safe for adults may be excessive for children. Although the testing data which the FDA receives are frequently ambiguous, the agency has neither the budget nor the staff to conduct its own testing program. Testing under the commission of the manufacturer can create conflicts of interest and encourage inaccurate, distorted, erroneous, and sometimes fraudulent safety data. Yet once an additive is approved, removal is a time-consuming and difficult process.

Since 1949, the FDA has had to ban at least two dozen widely used additives after new information showed them to be harmful. Every one of these substances was on an "approved" list when the bad news was discovered. Since 1980, an independent panel has been reviewing the safety of 415 additional GRAS additives. This review has not been completed, but the panel has identified a number of substances which need to be tested more thoroughly or restricted to some degree. It is virtually certain that some of the 3,000 or so additives now in common use will have to be banned one day.

Can Safety be Regulated?

The FDA is typical of the regulatory agencies which attempt to ensure food safety. For the most part, it is staffed by well-intentioned, dedicated, and capable people who want to do their jobs well. But there are practical limits to what any regulatory agency—whether it is the FDA, the EPA, the Department of Agriculture, the Federal Trade Commission, or any other—can accomplish.

Consumer advocates, industry spokesmen, independent research-ers, even some FDA scientists—nearly all complain that the FDA could do a better job. Some condemn the agency for being biassed; others, for being unscientific. Some say that the FDA needs more power; others, that it has too much already. Some argue that the agency is too sympathetic to the food industry; others that it pays too much attention to consumer critics. Each step the agency takes is virtually guaranteed to attract criticism from some sector. Pulled in many political, philosophic, and scientific directions and limited by budgetary, bureaucratic, legal, and policy constraints, the FDA pleases no one, perhaps because not even the FDA—an agency of the federal government with a staff of very highly trained experts—can fully make sense of food additives. Meanwhile, the FDA must attempt to carry out its responsibilities without conflicting with the many other agencies which claim regulatory authority.

The "Delaney Clause" of the 1958 Food Additives Amendment illustrates the FDA's dilemma. This clause states that no amount of any additive which causes cancer in animals or humans may be used in foods. It is based on the fact that we do not know how cancer is caused, so we cannot justify the intentional use of any carcinogenic substances in food. But loop-holes, technicalities, and politics have created exceptions. For example, the food industry has been able to persuade Congress that the medical and dietary benefits of saccharin outweigh its weak association with cancer. The FDA was able to remove this artificial sweetener from the GRAS list and to require the display of warnings on foods which contain the substance. But Congress has repeatedly prevented the agency from banning saccharin entirely. Similarly, the nitrites used to preserve processed meats can be converted, under certain heat or metabolic conditions, to nitrosamines, which are potent car-cinogens. Because nitrites probably do not, by themselves, cause cancer and because they do have unique benefits, the FDA con-tinues to sanction their use.

More recently, the food industry has complained, with some justification, that our ability to detect smaller and smaller amounts of cancer-causing substances has made the Delaney Clause an excessive burden. In sympathetic response, the Reagan Admin-istration brought political and bureaucratic pressure on the FDA to relax its standards. As a result, the FDA announced a new, *de minimus* rule which would allow minute residues of carcinogenic substances to remain in processed foods.

The FDA and other agencies are frequently hamstrung by political and ideological considerations. The Reagan Administration, which was unfriendly to most government regulation of business, acted as early as 1981 to limit the FDA's authority to issue many of the regulations which the agency itself considered necessary to carry out its responsibilities. When the administration reorganized the Public Health Service, it placed the FDA under the politically sensitive supervision of an Assistant Secretary of Health and Human Services. Meanwhile, even though the FDA already regulates products which take in one out of every four consumer dollars, Congress has continued to ask the agency to assume even more responsibilities. The result, according to a recent federal advisory committee, is an overwhelmed FDA that cannot deal effectively with the increased challenges brought on by the combination of traditional and new responsibilities.

Under the Bush Administration, the political climate has warmed slightly toward government action. A new reorganization promises to restore some of the agency's powers to enforce existing laws. A new, more energetic FDA commissioner has found sympathy in Congress for his pleas for more authority and a larger budget. A reinvigorated Federal Trade Commission has much more aggressively pursued misleading and deceptive food labeling. Whether this new activism can be sustained remains to be seen. But the important point is this: if politics and regulation cannot be separated, food safety may never be fully independent of politics and interest groups.

Chapter 2
Incidental Additives

Incidental additives are substances which become part of food without intentionally being added during the production process. This category includes all tested and approved additives in food-stuff used as ingredients in processed foods. But it also includes residues of pesticides, hormones, antibiotics, manufacturing and packaging chemicals, and other substances which enter the food anywhere between the field and the plate but serve no function in the final product.

Incidental additives, which normally appear only in trace amounts, are unavoidable side-effects of the modern food system. Most of them have not been adequately tested, and many have not been tested at all, so their safety is unknown. Incidental additives are truly hidden additives. Many are undetectable using current monitoring practices. Even when they can be identified, incidental additives do not need to be listed on product labels, so it is often impossible for the consumer to know when a food contains these forms of "unavoidable" contaminant.

Pesticides

Almost two billion pounds of pesticides are used annually to control insects, weeds, fungi, rodents, and other unwanted pests during crop production and storage. Made from approximately 1,800 different *active* and *inert* chemicals, these are powerful yet poorly tested compounds which are designed by definition to kill. An unknown number may cause a variety of health problems, including cancer, birth defects, mutations, miscarriages, nerve damage, and reproductive system damage. They are used primarily on produce, but pesticides may also contaminate meats, milk products, and ground water through the action of fog, wind, rain, and other, uncontrollable environmental factors. Pesticides may be even more concentrated in substances like cottonseed oil which are made from agricultural products not designated as food. Unfortunately, a substantial volume of pesticides is used simply for cosmetic purposes. A study released in March 1991, for example, reported that at least half of the pesticides applied to the citrus crop was used only to protect the appearance of the fruit.

The Environmental Protection Agency (EPA) is responsible for evaluating the testing of new pesticides, licensing their use, and setting maximum permissible levels for residues in food. Critics charge that the standards used by the EPA to make its decisions are distorted by faulty or simplistic assumptions, inadequate or falsified data, and political or subjective motives, and that the resulting tolerance levels are not realistic. Many agency insiders agree that the EPA could and should do a better job of regulating and controlling pesticide use. Industry and agency defenders reply that, in the absence of evidence that specific pesticides are harmful, these substances are needed to protect public health, increase harvest size, prevent loss during storage, and provide consumers with more nearly perfect produce. The benefits, they claim, outweigh the risks.

After the EPA has licensed a pesticide and issued standards for residues in food, the FDA becomes responsible for monitoring most industry compliance. Unfortunately, less than one percent of all food shipments is tested. A small but significant number of these tested samples normally reveal pesticide concentrations exceeding allowable tolerances. Unfortunately, by the time results have been obtained, the food from which the tested samples were taken has already been sold and consumed.

Even more disturbing to critics is the recent finding of the Office of Technology Assessment, a research arm of Congress, that the FDA's testing methods are able to detect only about half of the pesticides registered with the EPA. (The Department of Agriculture, which is responsible for monitoring pesticide residues in meat and milk products, can detect only about one pesticide in five.) Many of those which escape detection, moreover, may pose moderate to high threats to health. At least 45,000 cases of poisoning and 6,000 cancers are thought to be caused by pesticide exposure

Monitoring Pesticides

Pesticide manufacturers are required to advise the EPA whenever new tests are performed on pesticides. The EPA is then required to reevaluate and reregister pesticides in the light of the new information. This responsibility is not always carried out successfully. In 1991, a transportation accident spilled 19,000 gallons of the pesticide, metam-sodium, into the Sacramento River. Three weeks later, officials in California alerted residents of one nearby town that they had discovered studies in their files which indicated that metam-sodium, when combined with water, posed dangers of birth defects. Shortly thereafter, the EPA admitted that it had received the same "adverse effect" reports on the pesticide four years earlier. These reports had been filed and not even read until the accident called the agency's attention to the chemical. This was not an isolated incident. The EPA also admitted that studies warning about as many as 20 other chemicals had also been overlooked.

Some critics have charged that the studies in question had intentionally been buried by EPA officials who did not want to interfere with pesticide use. We will always have officials with axes to grind. But in fairness to the agency, the EPA suffers from many of the same problems as the FDA—bureaucratic inefficiencies, political pressures, budgetary deficiencies, policy limitations, etc. Nor is the agency immune from human error. Like most other regulatory agencies, the EPA is staffed by well-meaning, capable people who take their responsibilities seriously. We may simply be asking them to do more than anyone can reasonably expect them to do.

each year. No fewer than 27 of the pesticides approved by the EPA are thought to be potential carcinogens.

States also regulate the use of pesticides and other agricultural chemicals. But state regulation and enforcement is often spotty. States are allowed to impose more rigorous standards than those required by the federal government for foods grown or sold within their boundaries. But that by itself is no guarantee of effectiveness. In California, the nation's largest agricultural state, pesticides are regulated by the state Department of Agriculture, which is responsible both for promoting the agriculture industry and for protecting the public health. This creates a potential conflict of interest which critics claim is usually resolved in favor of agribusiness. Critics complain that far too many positions of leadership and influence within the department are appointed from the agriculture industry and that far too few spokesmen for other points of view are heard when important decisions are made.

Defenders of pesticides and other chemicals frequently call their critics "alarmists" and "toxic terrorists" who agitate public passions either to gain publicity or to impose Big Brother on the economy. They argue that trace residues of pesticides "pose no hazard to human health" and that the real danger in foods comes from toxins found naturally in foods and from the biological contamination which pesticides prevent. Chemical residues, they add, pose only negligible, theoretical hazards compared to the measurable risks associated with microbial contaminants or harmful, conscious behaviors like smoking and alcoholism. Pesticides, they conclude, are necessary weapons in the arsenal of agribusiness.

Pesticide use has increased ten times since the 1950s, partly because chemical-resistant pests have evolved; partly because agriculture has become increasingly dependent on chemicals; partly because federal produce standards, by assigning the highest grades to unblemished produce, actually encourage the application of pesticides; and partly because the food industry cannot afford even a single case of mishandling or contamination. Testing and monitoring methods have not kept pace with the explosive growth of pesticides. Promising testing methods are under development, but these may not become practical for years. Meanwhile, the volume and number of pesticides used both legally and illegally will continue to increase as pesticide use generates its own momentum.

It is not surprising that the FDA should refer to pesticide residues as "public worry number 1." Even while it downplays the magnitude of the problem, the agency's own figures underline the public's concern. Between 1982 and 1985, using admittedly inadequate monitoring methods, the FDA detected pesticide residues in almost half of 20,000 fruit and vegetable samples. The highest concentrations were found in produce grown in direct contact with the ground, such as celery, potatoes, and carrots. But residues were found most frequently in those fruits and vegetables which consumers insist be unblemished, such as strawberries, peaches, and bell peppers. Foreign-grown produce was much more likely to be contaminated than domestic produce. And foreign produce was also more likely to contain residues of pesticides and other chemicals which have been banned for use on domestic crops. Although only about one per cent of domestic samples exceeded tolerance levels, a substantial proportion of all domestic produce tested positive for pesticide residues.

Concern about pesticides continues to grow among consumers. A 1988 opinion poll commissioned by the Food Marketing Institute, a trade association of grocers, reported that seventy-five percent of consumers felt that pesticides and herbicides residues were a "serious problem." Another twenty percent considered residues to be "somewhat of a problem." In 1990, another Food Marketing Institute survey found that eighty percent of consumers thought that pesticides posed a serious health threat. Yet another survey reported that eighty-four percent of consumers would buy organic produce if it cost the same as nonorganic produce. When one major California grocery company recently asked a commercial testing service to inspect its produce, its sales of fruits and vegetables increased by a reported sixteen percent. Its subsequently sale of one million pounds of tested table grapes in one week at a price twenty cents higher than that of untested grapes was called "the largest single sale of produce in the history of the company."

The produce industry has indirectly acknowledged the depth of this consumer anxiety. In 1989, the industry launched a massive

Reducing Agricultural Chemicals

Farmers themselves are questioning whether or not the use of more and more agricultural chemicals is a good thing. In part, farmers have become concerned about their own exposure to these chemicals. In California, for example, farm workers have been required to wear protective outfits which resemble space suits when applying chemicals like the herbicide, Molinate, which is known to cause significant reproductive damage in small doses.

Consumer demand alone has stimulated a dramatic growth in the market for organic and natural foods. One authority recently estimated that the organic crop market would comprise as much as 10 percent of the national market by the year 1995. Growing numbers of farmers are complaining that pesticides simply do not work as well as they used to. Many farmers who are not moving toward natural production are employing non-chemical techniques and using fewer agricultural chemicals in attempts to use chemicals only when the need exists.

public relations campaign to encourage greater public acceptance of pesticides. In 1990, the agribusiness community organized the "FoodWatch" program to defend the industry's position aggressively. Sponsored by a major industry organization and funded by chemical companies and trade groups, this campaign attempted to answer criticisms about pesticides and to promote pesticide use and the industry in general.

Hormones and Steroids

Other residues are left by chemicals which are used on the modern, biotechnological farm. Natural, synthetic, and genetically engineered hormones and anabolic steroids are used to lower production costs by accelerating the growth of animals prior to slaughter or to increase the volume of milk that animals are able to produce. These substances may increase production, but they may also have other, unintended effects. Critics charge that the nutritional quality of milk produced by cows injected with bovine growth hormone, for example, may be changed for the worse. Many treated animals, moreover, suffer from infections more often, leading to even more widespread use of antibiotics (see below). Finally, the difficulty of policing the use of these substances, which are frequently bought without prescriptions, may make hormone abuse more dangerous, if not more likely.

Federal officials assure the public that minute levels of contamination pose no health risk. Because most of the hormones currently used are "natural" substances presumably used in very small amounts, they should be fully metabolized by the animals if sufficient time is allowed between dosage and slaughter. In reality, however, this does not always happen. Diethylstilbestrol (DES), for example, a synthetic hormone similar to the natural female hormone, estrogen, has caused cancer among the offspring of human women who were given minute amounts of the chemical during pregnancy. It was formerly used to fatten beef, but its use was banned in 1979 after hormone residues were found in meat treated up to a week before slaughter. Other synthetic hormones used in beef and chicken have been associated with a condition known as *thelarche*, or *precocious puberty*, in which children's reproductive organs develop at very early ages. Hormone

Bovine Somatotropin

One hormone which has received considerable attention in recent years is Bovine Somatotropin (BST), or Bovine Growth Hormone (BGH). The use of BST, a synthetic version of a naturally occuring hormone, reportedly can increase milk production by up to thirty percent. Milk from treated cows has been under testing since the middle of the last decade, and this milk has been allowed to be introduced into the national milk supply.

Representatives of the food industry have supported the use of growth hormone as safe and useful. Preliminary studies released by the FDA tended to support the industry's claims. Even the influential journal, **Science**, published an editorial supporting the use of BGH and criticizing opponents of the hormone as rabble rousers who sought to use "safety and health issues as a red herring to strengthen their economic concerns." In Spring 1991, a panel of scientists at the National Institutes of Health (NIH) gave BST a controversial nod of approval.

Despite these reassurances, a number of authorities have raised important questions about the safety of this genetically engineered hormone and about the general wisdom of its use. Charging that the nutritional value of treated milk is affected, critics argue that BST, by increasing the fat content of milk, may increase the threat from other contaminants and cause herds to suffer additional health problems. Despite the NIH panel's findings, opponents continue to insist that not enough is known about the effects of BGH on infants and children. Finally, farm economists claim that BGH is not needed at a time when milk surplusses exist and that the real victims will be the small farmers who will be hurt most by declining milk prices.

use is so controversial that the European Community, responding to pressure from European consumers, voted in 1988 to ban the importation of hormone-laden American beef.

Antibiotics

Half of all antibiotics used in the United States are administered to food animals. Recent estimates are that up to 90% of chickens, 80% of pigs, and 60% of beef receive routine, sub-therapeutic doses in their feed. Livestock crowding on "factory farms" and feed lots creates ideal conditions for the spread of disease among farm

animals. Antibiotics are used because such microbiological contamination could jeopardize the health and marketability of food
animals. Antibiotics offer secondary benefits because they also
increase growth rates and litter sizes, toughen egg shells, and
reduce production costs.

Antibiotics have not been totally successful in preventing
microbial contamination. In fact, the use of antibiotics is thought
to have encouraged the development of new strains of bacteria
which are resistant to the antibiotics. Bacterial contamination of
poultry, for example, has significantly increased during the last
decade despite the mounting use of antibiotics. Recent studies have
estimated that up to 50% of retail chickens have been contaminated
by salmonella bacteria.

Even when used with proper controls, antibiotic residues in
meats and poultry may cause allergies and other health problems
for those who are sensitive to the chemicals which make up the
drugs and pose unknown risks for others. And antibiotics are not

Testing for Antibiotics

Testing for antibiotic residues in foods leaves much to be desired. More
than 20,000 different drugs are used for veterinary purposes. Yet until
recently, the FDA has done little if any routine testing except for specific
chemicals. One recent critic estimated that the tests run on meat are able to
detect, at best, 6,000 of the 20,000 drugs currently used for veterinary
purposes. The FDA itself hardly inspires unquestioned confidence. In 1989
and 1990, the agency ran three different tests on the same samples of milk
to determine the extent to which residues of sulfa drugs remained. Each test
provided different results. In February 1990, the FDA accepted the results of
the least sensitive of these tests to declare that a dramatic reduction in
antibiotic contamination had occurred during the previous two years. Two
months later, the FDA announced that its conclusions had been premature.
Admitting that trace residues were found in fifty of seventy samples tested,
the agency insisted that the extent of contamination posed no health hazard.
The report downplayed the facts that residues were found, that tests were not
performed to identify residues of many other potential drugs, and that the
illegal use of these and other drugs may well be widespread. (This may be a
particularly thorny problem for milk, because a single carton conceivably
contains milk from thousands of cows.)

always used legally, particularly when they are frequently available over-the-counter without prescription. Sulfamethazine, for example, is an antibiotic added to animal feed in order to prevent respiratory illness among cattle, pork, and poultry. Even though it is banned for use in milk-producing animals, residues of this cancer-causing and allergenic drug were found in seventy-three percent of milk samples taken in 10 major American cities in 1988.

In November 1990, the General Accounting Office (GAO) criticized the FDA's antibiotic testing program. It pointed out that the FDA failed to determine the extent to which drugs given dairy cows contaminated the food supply, failed to inquire into the actual safety of the drugs which did leave residues, failed to use adequate milk samples, failed to test for at least half the drugs used by dairy farmers, and failed to resolve contradictory results of laboratory tests. An FDA spokesman admitted that its testing was not adequate but complained that the agency simply lacked the budget to perform the tests as thoroughly as the GAO would have liked.

Packaging Chemicals

Another source of incidental contamination is food packaging. Through simple contact, chemicals used in the manufacture of food containers may be absorbed by the foods within the package. Lead, for example, can leech into food from the leaded solder used in certain cans. Plastics are troublesome because of the chemicals used during the manufacture of plastic containers. Even paper cartons can pose problems because they may contain residues of dangerous manufacturing chemicals and by-products like PCBs, dioxin, and formaldehyde. An additional source of concern is the aluminum used in cans and cartons, because aluminum has been ambiguously connected to dementia-type disorders like Alzheimer's Disease.

Chemicals in "microwave-ready" packages may have additional, unknown consequences, because the microwave oven can raise temperatures high enough to vaporize some of the chemicals. The FDA recently questioned whether or not some of the "browning" or "crisping" devices known as "heat susceptors" might not disintegrate under the high temperatures produced by the microwaves and migrate into foods, particularly foods with high fat contents. Admitting that the possibility of migration had taken it by surprise, the agency expressed the additional concern that the chemical components of adhesives, paper, paperboard, plastics, and other packaging material may be migrating as well.

Other chemicals

A number of other sources may introduce incidental additives into food. Less has been written about these contaminants, which may include trace residues of any chemical indirectly used in any phase of food production. Extremely small amounts of chemicals used in fertilizers, lubricants, cleansers, solvents, dyes, paints, waxes, shellacs, etc. may be found in the food supply. So, too, may industrial contaminants, such as mercury, lead, PCBs, dioxin, and illegally dumped chemicals, as well as unapproved or banned pesticides, like DDT, dieldrin, and endrin; and industrial or agricultural wastes. Many of these chemicals are not considered additives, but they are unavoidable byproducts of an increasingly technological system of food production and distribution.

The contamination of water is a particular problem because of the central importance water has for all life. More than seventy billion gallons of hazardous wastes are dumped into landfills and water annually. And this does not take into account the wastes and other hazardous material which accidentally leak into the environment. These chemicals contaminate drinking water, work their way into plants and animals which consume contaminated water,

Contamination of Meats

Because both animal feed and groundwater are subject to contamination, meats may actually contain a greater variety of pesticides and other chemicals than fruits or vegetables. This is not just true of farm animals. Recent studies have found extensive contamination from a number of sources in fish and seafood as well. Fish taken from selected inland areas such as the Great Lakes tend to be highly contaminated.

Animals tend to store contaminants in their fats, so fatty meats, fish, and seafood are likely to be more hazardous than leaner ones. Particular care should be taken with foods packed in their own oil, such as tuna fish, sardines, and mackerel.

and build up in significant concentrations in fish, shellfish, and other animals which consume large amounts of water or organisms which live in water.

One chemical which received considerable recent attention is Alar (daminozide). The use of this "growth regulator" illustrates some of the problems associated with chemical-intensive agriculture. Often erroneously referred to as a pesticide, Alar was used to slow the ripening process and minimize crop losses in apples as well as some other fruits, vegetables, and peanuts. Alar is absorbed by the produce, so residues were found in apple sauce, peanut butter, fruit juices, and other foods made from Alar-treated crops. These are all foods which are frequently consumed in proportionally large amounts by children, who tend to have much lower resistance to the effects of chemicals.

When the EPA uncovered evidence that Alar might cause cancer, it initiated the slow and tedious process of removing approval from the chemical. The EPA cannot legally suspend a product unless it can demonstrate that the product threatens the public with an "imminent hazard." Nevertheless, in response to consumer pressure, many food markets chose not to sell fruits treated with daminozide, and most food producers attempted to eliminate raw materials exposed to Alar from their products. In 1989, Uniroyal Chemical Company, the manufacturer of Alar, announced that it was voluntarily suspending production of the chemical in response to the public concern about its safety.

The banning of Alar did not undo the exposure which had occurred since the chemical was first introduced in the early 1970s. Alar may not even have been necessary. Apple growers protested that banning the use of Alar would bring catastrophe to the industry. Nevertheless, except for a momentary dip in apple sales during the Alar controversy, sales quickly rebounded to pre-controversy levels. With virtually no long-range sales drop off, the loss of Alar proved not to be a major problem for the industry.

(Ironically, the Alar episode may have encouraged the increased use of chemicals in agriculture. Consumer reluctance to buy apples created a temporary depression in the apple market. While momentary, this was sufficient to drive a number of small apple farmers, including many who never used Alar at all, out of business. Apple growing, as a consequence, became dominated even more by larger companies which were more likely to use chemical-intensive methods of production.)

Irradiation

Legally defined as an additive, irradiation is a relatively new process of exposing food to high energy radiation. It is slowly finding a place in the arsenal of food technology. At present, its uses are limited to killing insects or microbes in fruits and vegetables, wheat, wheat flour, spices, herbs, and powders; preventing potatoes from sprouting; and killing *trichinella* worms in pork and salmonella and other bacteria in poultry. Consumer resistance and state regulatory restrictions have dampened the industry's eagerness to use irradiation techniques more extensively. Nevertheless, government regulators are gradually expanding the legal applications of the technology. Irradiation will certainly be used more widely in the future to control pests, prolong shelf life, preserve quality, or modify the characteristics of food.

Irradiation has its drawbacks. Food is not always as wholesome or nutritious after irradiation, which destroys vitamins and minerals. In some cases, food characteristics like texture or taste are changed for the worse. Irradiation does not produce radioactive food, but irradiated food has been linked in inconsistent and often contradictory tests to a number of health problems, including cancer and chromosome damage. Critics have also objected that the "unique radiolytic products" and "free radicals" created by the irradiation of food may be harmful. Irradiation, finally, may not be necessary. Less invasive handling and processing techniques can accomplish many of the same results.

Irradiation may also be the most hidden of additives. Labels of irradiated food are legally required to display a "Radura" emblem, which resembles a flower encircled by a thick, broken line. But no indication is required when irradiated ingredients are used in non-irradiated food. Moreover, irradiation can easily be abused. There is no way to determine whether or how often a food has been irradiated or how large a dose it has received. Irradiation has already been used illegally to "freshen" rancid meats in Europe, killing offensive bacteria but leaving behind the toxic wastes which the bacteria had previously produced.

Foods of the Future

The test tube is becoming an important factor in the food system. For generations, farmers and scientists have employed techniques like cross-breeding in order to achieve certain desired qualities. But the growing ability to manipulate genetic structures of foods and other substances has enabled the food industry to shorten the periods of experimentation, control the outcomes more predictably, and create products which might not have been created by cross-breeding alone.

The public is not entirely comfortable with genetic engineering. The food industry is trying very hard to encourage the public's willingness to accept this technology. One of the most important but unspoken undercurrents in the controversy over bovine somatotropin (see the sidebar on page 21) has been the symbolic significance of the outcome. Both the food industry and its critics are very much aware that the public's acceptance of this particular hormone will do much to assure the future development and use of genetically engineered products.

The argument over genetic engineering may in fact be over, regardless of the outcome of the bovine somatotropin debate. Genetically enhanced food and non-food products are already in the marketplace, and increasing numbers will be added in the future. New, genetically modified means of pest control, for example, are being developed to take the place of chemical pesticides. New strains of crops are being engineered to have enhanced nutritional, aesthetic, or cosmetic qualities; to resist specific pests or specific agricultural chemicals; and even to be partially self-fertilizing. Research is under way to design meats which are lower in fat or cholesterol and higher in protein. And genetically engineered medical and pharmaceutical products have been available for several years.

Other developments can also be expected. "Engineered" and "designer foods" already take up grocery-store shelf space. Increasing numbers will appear in the future. These foods are developed to solve specific problems or achieve specific goals. While they often do this successfully, they may also cause additional problems. For example, "restructured" meats which are sold as "light" or "lower in calories" may actually be higher in salt, MSG, and other chemicals. Fat substitutes made from egg and milk protein, sucrose polyesters, modified fatty acids, grains, or other substances may be used in commercial and nutritionally empty foods which contain substantial amounts of other chemicals and additives. Sales of these foods may also encourage consumers to eat fewer fruits and vegetables and to believe that reducing fats, calories, and cholesterol is all that is needed for a healthy diet.

No one really knows what all these new foods will mean for food safety. Items which are entirely new will be rigorously tested, so they will probably be safe for most people. But there can never be guarantees, particularly when the food item is so new that we have no long-term experience with its effects. Consumers of the future will need to continue being discriminating about the food they eat.

Chapter 3
Natural Contaminants

Natural contaminants include any number of bacteria, fungi, worms, molds, parasites, and other microorganisms. They have always compromised the safety of food, and presumably they will continue to affect the foods we eat for the foreseeable future. Human carelessness intensifies the effects of these hazards, but even the most careful handling and processing may be insufficient to ward them off entirely.

In contrast to chemical contamination, natural contaminants generally work quickly. Still, consumers may not always be aware that their food has been contaminated. In fact, health experts estimate that consumers are actually less informed about food contamination today than they were only five years ago. Food poisonings have increased significantly in recent years. Yet many people simply accept them as ordinary stomach upset. It has been estimated that as many as 10,000 people die each year from food-borne disease. Exposure is a particular problem for the young, the elderly, the sick, and those with immune systems which have already been compromised.

A partial list of natural contaminants might include:

AFLATOXIN, a natural mold found in nuts, peanuts, grains, and corn, which can also be contracted from the meat and dairy products of animals which have consumed aflatoxin-contaminated feed. Aflatoxin is thought to cause liver cancer.

BOTULINUM (Clostridium botulinum), an *anaerobic* bacteria (one which grows without oxygen) which, spread through improper canning and preparation, causes botulism. Although rare, botulism can be fatal. Its symptoms include nerve and vision problems as well as fatigue.

CAMPYLOBACTER, which is usually spread from fecal contact during the slaughter or processing of meats, poultry, and dairy products. Up to two million cases of campylobacter poisoning may occur annually. Its symptoms include severe stomach inflammation and diarrhea.

CHOLERA, which is spread largely by contact with infected fecal matter in water or sewage. Its symptoms include diarrhea, cramps, vomiting, and dehydration. It is extremely rare in the United States and usually contracted by eating raw or undercooked shellfish. Cholera is easily cured, but it can be fatal if left untreated.

CIGUATERA, a form of food poisoning caused by eating contaminated fish such as red snapper. It can produce fever, breathing difficulties, chills, or nerve irregularities.

ESCHERICHIA COLI (E. coli), a common cause of intestinal upset and diarrhea among the young and among those who are travelling. It is not normally serious, although at least one rare strain may be quite severe. E. coli is normally associated with meat and dairy products.

HEPATITIS, a virus causing an inflammation of the liver and general flu-like symptoms, which is spread largely through contact with fecal matter and through careless food handling by someone already infected with the virus. Hepatitis can be fatal, though more frequently it causes prolonged liver weakness.

LISTERIA, another anaerobic bacteria often spread through improper handling and processing of some meats and dairy products like soft cheese. Listeria can be fatal for up to twenty-five percent of the young, the aged, and the infirm, though for most others the symptoms resemble a mild flu. Listeria can also contribute to the incubation of encephalitis and meningitis. This is a relatively newly discovered bacteria, the first major outbreak of which in 1985 resulted in at least forty-eight deaths.

PARALYTIC SHELLFISH POISONING, a serious food poisoning caused generally by an organism found in shellfish from restricted and "red tide" areas. Paralytic shellfish poisoning can cause dizziness, breathing problems, nausea, and loss of coordination.

PERFRIGENS, a bacteria normally found in stews, gravies, and other dishes which are allowed to sit at room temperature or higher for extended periods. While rarely fatal, it can produce uncomfortable gas pains and diarrhea.

SALMONELLA, a group of bacteria which may be found in eggs, poultry, pork, red meats, dairy products, seafood, and products which contain them. It has also been found recently in pre-cut melons. Salmonella is the leading cause of food-borne illness in the United States, responsible for up to four million cases of food poisoning yearly. It is characterized by intestinal inflammation accompanied by cramps, diarrhea, and nausea lasting up to a week.

SCOMBROID FISH POISONING, which is a mild but uncomfortable food poisoning caused by a toxin produced when fish like tuna and mackerel spoil. It causes an allergic reaction which may include dizziness, muscular weakness, thirst, and heart palpitations.

STAPHYLOCOCCUS, a bacteria which grows rapidly and is spread almost exclusively by careless handling. It can produce diarrhea and nausea. Staphylococcus contamination occurs most often in processed meat, dairy, and prepared starchy dishes.

TOXOPLASMOSIS, which is a parasite spread mainly from cats to animals and humans, almost always by human carelessness. It can cause particular problems for fetuses exposed from foods consumed by their mothers.

TRICHINOSIS, which is caused by consuming meats such as wild game and pork which contain the *trichinella* worm. Its symptoms include muscle pain, fever, and water retention.

Today as in the past, natural contamination often results from careless growing conditions and improper storage or preparation by the end consumer. But the modern food system has added numerous other sources of contamination. Factory farms, dairies, hatcheries, and eggeries create crowded conditions which are ideal for the spread of bacteria. Inadequate inspection allows healthy animals to come in contact with unhealthy ones. Transportation,

HUMAN ERROR

A 1991 outbreak of cholera illustates the central role human error plays in the spread of bacteria. Contaminated crab meat which had been processed and cooked in the South American country of Ecuador was put into plastic bags and flown to the United States. Even though cholera had already reached the epidemic proportions in Ecuador, neither customs agents nor food inspectors examined the shipment. The tainted seafood was then served, without even being reheated, to unsuspecting diners in New Jersey, eight of whom contracted the rare yet potentially fatal disease.

slaughter, processing, and handling create additional opportunities for the spread of microbiological and organic contaminants and favorable conditions for their growth. Inadequate temperature controls and unsanitary machinery, equipment, and working conditions can foster still more bacterial growth.

The food industry claims that it can minimize the impact of these contaminants through the use of chemicals like pesticides and fungicides and processes like vacuum packaging and irradiation. Critics are not convinced. Up to sixty percent of retail meats may be contaminated, along with a substantial portion of dairy products and eggs. Salmonella and campylobacter contamination of eggs and chickens alone has mushroomed during the last few years of increasingly intense chemical use.

Natural contamination is a growing problem which can be magnified by good intentions. Attempting to cut down on cholesterol and fats, many consumers have turned away from red meats and begun selecting poultry and seafoods instead. The resulting increase in demand has placed impossible new demands on an already overworked monitoring and inspection system for poultry and a virtually nonexistent system for seafood and fish.

Chapter 4
Additives And You

Consumers must make up their own minds about additives in their food. One consumer may absolutely refuse to eat anything which contains even a hint of technology. Another consumer may value time, convenience, and ease so much as to trust the food industry and government regulators unquestioningly. Between these extremes lie any number of intermediate positions.

We consumers must take the initiative and make choices we can live with. After all, we make choices which affect our health and safety every day. We choose whether or not to smoke, to drink, to climb mountains, to run stop signs, even to use illegal drugs. Why stop there? Other choices will be made, by us if we take the initiative or by someone else if we do not.

Avoiding all food additives may not be necessary. But, as a personal recommendation, it may be good judgment to reduce consumption of these chemicals as far as possible. After hours of hearings, the Senate Select Committee on Nutrition recommended exactly that. Most nutritionists and independent observers of food technology also endorse this recommendation. Even if for no other reason, minimizing exposure to additives will also minimize exposure to those high-fat, high-sodium, low-nutrition "junk foods" in which additives are so commonly used.

How to Choose Food Wisely

Keep things in perspective. Don't worry excessively over the safety of the food you are eating. We possess remarkably efficient immune and detoxifying systems which have evolved over thousands of generations in the face of countless natural and man-made hazards. We may not have biological experience with many of the new chemicals found in modern foods, but we have developed very effective mechanisms to foster immunities and protect the body. This does not mean that we can abandon all precautions. But we can expect to withstand certain amounts of exotic chemicals. Unless you have a defective immunological system or some other debilitating condition, excessive worry about what might be in your food may be more harmful than an occasional indulgence or indiscretion. Individual food items are far less significant an influence on health than your overall diet and lifestyle. Good health certainly lies more in the direction of a balanced life, intelligent eating habits, adequate sleep, and moderate exercise.

Know about the foods you are buying. The number of chemicals used in foods will continue to grow. It may not be possible to avoid all exposure to these substances, but it is a good idea to stay informed about the food you buy. Use this guide to help you learn about the foods you have bought and those you will buy in the future.

At the same time, find out more about these substances. A guide of this size cannot begin to summarize everything there is to know. Research continues to reveal previously unknown benefits and risks of additives. New additives are routinely being introduced. Keep up to date about these recent developments. Your local newspaper and even radio and television news and information broadcasts will keep you informed about the more dramatic developments. The last section of this guide is a carefully selected list of current and dependable sources of additional information.

Use Common Sense. Choose a "better-safe-than-sorry" attitude. There are only two general types of "mistakes" you can make regarding food safety. First, you can assume that a food is safe when it is really harmful. Or you can assume that it is harmful when it is really safe. Consider which of these "mistakes" is easier for you to live with.

When in doubt, assume that something is harmful even if it is actually safe. If a food looks, smells, or tastes odd, don't eat it. If a product is past its shelf-date, don't buy it. If a package is broken or a can is dented, pick another one that is intact. If plastic from a package melts over the food in your microwave, throw the food out and start over. If an egg is broken in the carton, don't add it to your omelet.

Opportunities to exercise common sense occur every day. The important thing is to act. Think about the potential consequences of your decision, and act accordingly. Don't fall victim to the "famous-last-words" phenomenon.

Read food labels.   These may not tell you everything you want to know, but labels do give you certain basic pieces of information. For most foods, labels will list the intentional ingredients in descending order by weight. In addition, labels may also include nutritional information such as vitamin and sodium content or the number of calories per serving. They will seldom tell you which specific spice, food color, food flavor, or vegetable oil is used in the food, and you may have to add up all the separate types of sugar. But most of the time the label will tell you that the food does or does not contain these substances. Labels will not necessarily provide safety information or storage and handling recommendations, but they will include any legally required health warnings. If nothing else, labels will at least allow you to compare brands for the types of ingredients and additives they contain.

Unfortunately, you cannot depend totally on labels. Certain ingredients will not be listed at all. GRAS additives, incidental additives, and additives used by suppliers of ingredients but not by the final manufacturer do not need to be included. Except for colors and flavors, labels seldom indicate whether an additive is natural or artificial. Some foods have been exempted from labelling requirements entirely. Any labelling on meats or produce will be totally voluntary. Until recently, labels on foods prepared according to "standard recipes" needed only identify the name of the food. These standard recipes are legal "Standards of Identity" which define "generic" formulas for 235 different types of processed food. Foods normally produced according to standard recipes include dairy products, pasta, baked goods, mayonnaise, canned fruits and vegetables, margarine, peanut butter, soft drinks, jellies, etc. Labels on these foods must now include listings of ingredients.

Remember that labels are also used to sell the product. Be skeptical about the claims they make. Nutritional claims on the packaging must be at least partially documented on the label, but other claims may not be regulated. The term *natural*, for example, has had no legal meaning (unless it referred to meat or poultry). It was frequently used as a marketing gimmick. Many consumers, assuming that natural is more nutritious than artificial, have been willing to spend more for a product claiming to be "natural." (On the other hand, the term *organic* may have more legal meaning, because some states have acted to give it legal definition. The Nutrition Labeling and Education Act of 1990 gives a federal definition of the term, effective as of 1993.) *Enriched* tells you that some of the nutrients which were destroyed during processing have been replaced. *Fortified* means that some vitamins and minerals not normally found in the food have been added. Other potentially misleading terms have been used, including *real, pure, fresh, light* or *lite,* and other words or phrases which have seldom if ever been given legal enforcement or even legal definition. Other equally meaningless claims have included *no added sugar, no preservatives added, fiber-rich, fat-free, no cholesterol,* and similar statements which have encouraged consumers to draw some conclusion about the food they have bought.

Labels must be truthful, but they can tell the truth very creatively. Claims about fat content, serving sizes, nutritional benefits, and the like may be questionable or meaningless. Even product names and label design may be designed to present products in the most positive light without running afoul of regulatory standards. New legislation, new regulations, and, recently, more aggressive enforcement of existing laws by the FDA and other state and national agencies may help eliminate some of the more obvious shortcomings. But no amount of regulation can take the place of informed consumer behavior.

Avoid highly processed and refined foods. Prepackaged, precooked, frozen, instant, or imitation foods, artificial "substitutes," prepared mixes, "snack foods," and "junk foods" are the largest single sources of both intentional and incidental food additives in the modern diet. These mass-produced and highly advertised products are quite likely to contain troublesome additives. They are much more likely to contain the saturated fats, salts, and sugars that so many nutritionists regard as dietary time bombs. They are also subject to much more handling, which increases the possibility of accidental contamination.

Avoid particularly troublesome additives. Different authorities will offer different lists of additives to avoid. But most will include some or all of the following chemicals (all of which are described in the dictionary part of this guide):

Aluminum compounds	MSG and other **glutamates**
Artificial colors	Nitrates
Artificial flavors	Nitrites
Artificial sweeteners	Propyl gallate
BHA	Quinine
BHT	Sodium chloride (salt)
Brominated vegetable oil	Sulfites

Your own list of additives to avoid might include other substances as well, depending on your own personal experiences. A later section of this guide lists foods which are likely to contain these and other questionable additives.

Include more fresh foods in your diet. "Whole" foods—fresh fruits and vegetables, whole grains, whole-grain products, etc.—seldom contain additives. Frozen fruits and vegetables will expose you to fewer additives than canned. Fresh cuts of meat from a butcher will contain fewer additives than canned, packaged, or "imitation" meats. There are always exceptions to this rule. But as a rule, the closer a food is to its natural state, the less likely it is to contain additives.

Shop for and prepare fresh fruits and vegetables carefully to protect yourself from incidental additives. If possible, buy groceries from reputable organic sources or from grocers who can certify that their produce is free of agricultural chemicals. Look for locally

FOODS MOST LIKELY TO CONTAIN CONTAMINANTS

A recent study listed some of the foods most likely to contain some form of contamination. The list included **apples, beans, beef, carrots, chicken, corn, grapes, lettuce, oranges, peaches, pork, potatoes, soybeans, tomatoes,** and **wheat**. Other recent studies have pointed to the extreme risks of contamination from **shellfish,** particularly from mollusks like **clams** and **oysters.**

The importance of finding a dependable supplier of safe and healthy foods is all the more important because these are some of the most widely consumed food items in the modern diet.

grown fruits and vegetables which are less likely to contain residues of agricultural chemicals. Be skeptical about perfect-looking produce. It may owe its looks to pesticides. Washing produce carefully, perhaps with a mild solution of dish detergent and water, will remove some but not all pesticide residues. Peeling will remove more (as well as many of the nutrients). Look for meat and poultry that have been grown without the use of hormones, antibiotics, or treated feeds. Meats imported from Australia or New Zealand, for example, are more likely to be hormone-free. For greater protection from packaging material, buy supplies in bulk or in glass containers. If you can, avoid buying foods in plastic or aluminum containers, and make a particular point to avoid cooking plastic-wrapped foods in microwave ovens.

Eat a variety of foods. Avoid the overconsumption of only a few types of foods in order to reduce your exposure to any single additive or group of additives. Many chemicals tend to concentrate in certain parts of the body. Variety in the diet will reduce the possibility of individual chemicals becoming concentrated at potentially harmful levels. Finally, variety offers the added psychological advantage of making all food more interesting and tasteful.

Reduce the amount of fat and oil in your diet. Cutting down on fat and oil makes good nutritional sense. Study after study has concluded that fats, and particularly animal and dairy fats, cause weight problems and contribute to cholesterol problems. What is more, most animals store residues of pesticides, herbicides, and other chemicals in their fat. When meat animals, poultry, or fish consume tainted food or water, residues of these contaminants are likely to build up in fatty tissues through a process known as *bioconcentration*. Likewise, when crops are sprayed with pesticides or other agricultural chemicals, any residues which remain are likely to be concentrated in the oils and seeds. Steps like reducing your consumption of meats and fats, buying foods with lower levels of fats and oils, trimming visible fat from meats, removing skin from fish and poultry, buying low-fat or non-fat milk products, and consuming oils from crops grown specifically as foods (such as olive or safflower oil) will help minimize exposure to contaminants.

Select, handle, prepare, and store food wisely. Even though biological contaminants exist naturally, the human hand is the single most important factor in preventing or encouraging their spread. Regardless of the efforts made by the food industry and government agencies, much of the responsibility must rest on the consumer. Fortunately, the consumer *can* make a difference simply by taking a few basic precautions.

Examine foods carefully in the store. Buying as fresh as possible may not prevent you from purchasing meats or prepared foods which are already contaminated, but it will help assure that the growth of any bacteria or other contaminants is minimized. Examine foods for odd colors, smells, or textures, and avoid those with visible fungi or molds. Make sure that the food you purchase has been shelved or refrigerated properly in the store. Pay attention to "sell by" dates on packages.

Store foods properly at home to minimize contamination. Refrigerate foods which need to be refrigerated using containers which are designed for food storage. Some contaminants, including listeria and yersinia, can actually grow under refrigeration, but many others will be prevented or arrested. Don't expect refrigeration to work miracles. It will not prevent decay, so eat stored food within a reasonable time. Don't take unnecessary chances. If stored food does not seem right, throw it out.

Prepare foods carefully. Make sure your hands, your tools, and your work surfaces are kept clean. The possibility of cross-contamination is frequently overlooked, so make sure that potentially contaminated pieces and juices do not come in contact with other food items. Cook foods thoroughly. Most biological contaminants will be killed if food is exposed to sufficient cooking temperatures. Be cautious about cooking in microwaves, which may not heat uniformly enough to kill all contaminants.

Meats deserve special attention. Organ meats like liver, kidney, and heart may contain particularly high concentrations of cholesterol and incidental contaminants. Eat these in moderation. The high temperatures associated with grilling, broiling, or frying muscle meats like steaks, ribs, and roasts can produce *heterocyclic aromatic amines*, which are strongly suspected of causing cancer. Where possible, cook muscle meats under lower temperatures and for shorter periods of time. You might even precook muscle meats in a microwave to lessen the amount of heat and cooking time needed. And always purchase meats from a trustworthy source.

Know yourself and those who depend on you. Many people are sensitive to specific foods. Reactions to food may include the simple, behavioral change that follows excessive sugar consumption as well as the much more complex physiological changes that are caused by serious chemical or enzyme imbalances. Perhaps as many as one person in six is allergic to some food item. Reactions can range from mild lethargy, headache, runny nose, or rash to severe stomach upset, breathing difficulties, anaphylactic shock, and even death. Many additives are made from substances which cause allergic reactions, and other additives can be allergenic by themselves. Certain foods, such as cow's milk, eggs, wheat, soy, corn, and nuts, are particularly allergenic. And certain people—infants, pregnant women, the elderly, and the infirm—are likely to be more sensitive to the effects of specific chemicals. But any given individual may have a personal reaction or allergy to almost any food.

Pay attention to your aesthetic reactions as well. For examples: How does processed food really taste? What is the aftertaste of nondairy creamer? How does imitation chocolate "feel" in your mouth? How do artificial flavors compare to real flavors? How long does a brand of salad dressing continue to taste exciting? After how many meals does a specific frozen entree become boring? In short, how satisfied do you feel when you have finished eating? One of the most convincing reasons to avoid additives is the extra enjoyment that comes from eating the "real" foods that the food processing industry is trying to imitate.

Be a squeaky wheel. Make your desires known to your local grocer. Ask the store manager to stock the kinds of food you want to buy. Be willing to shop elsewhere if your concerns are not heard. Join and support consumer organizations, such as those included in the bibliography, which can command the attention of government and industry. Write letters. Let your representatives in the state and federal governments hear from you so that they know what issues their constituents feel strongly enough about to write. Communicate with the regulatory agencies—the FDA, the EPA, and the USDA. These may be parts of the bureaucracy, but they are not independent of citizen pressure. Indeed, agency officials have become increasingly sensitive to the growing consumer demand for more effective regulation. Write food manufacturers themselves to express your dissatisfaction with and especially your appreciation of their food products. Food companies, after all, are profit-seeking institutions which cannot afford to become alienated from their customers. Finally, express yourself through your spending. Consider your purchases to be reflections of your personal approval. You do not have to buy any product which fails to measure up to your own standards of acceptability. At the same time, your dollars will encourage grocers and food manufacturers to continue offering the types of foods you approve of.

Put your mouth where your money is. Once you have found a store which responds to your needs and wants, shop there. Store owners are entirely justified when they complain about consumers who demand certain foods but then refuse to buy them once the requested items are in stock. Additive-free foods may cost a little more, and the markets which sell them may not be conveniently located. But if you want these markets to exist, you need to support them. By patronizing stores which are sensitive to your needs, you can help guarantee that the foods you want will be available the next time you shop. It does make a difference.

Chapter 5
How Additives Are Used

ACIDIFIERS (Acidulants, acidifying agents) control the acidity of processed foods, make dough rise, or change the flavor or tartness of various foods. Some are also used as preservatives or antibrowning agents. Look for acidifiers like benzoic acid or citric acid in soft drinks, jelly, desserts, candy, cheese and cheese spreads, baked goods, frozen deserts, etc. As acids, all can erode tooth enamel and cause cavities.

ALKALIES (pH adjusting agents, bases) such as sodium hydroxide act as preservatives or flavor improvers by reducing the acidity or controlling the alkalinity (opposite of acidity) of foods like dairy products, canned vegetables, tomato products, chocolate, olives, baked goods, frozen desserts, etc.

ANTIBROWNING AGENTS, including various sulfite compounds, prevent cut fruits and vegetables from becoming oxidized and turning brown. (See antioxidants.) A small number of people are known to be highly allergic to sulfites in particular.

ANTICAKING AGENTS such as silicates prevent powders like salt, seasoned salt, baking powder, nondairy creamer, and soft drink powder from absorbing water and becoming hard.

ANTIFOAMING AGENTS (defoaming agents) prevent liquids from foaming. Silicones and other antifoaming agents are found in fruit juices, wine, beer, coffee creamer, jelly, milk products, baked goods, etc. Some antifoaming agents can be toxic in extremely large doses.

ANTIMYCOTIC AGENTS (antimold agents, antirope agents, mold inhibitors, mold or rope retarders) prevent the growth of molds, bacteria, and other microorganisms in bread, baked goods, cheese, processed meats, syrup, jelly, dried fruit, etc. Common antimycotic agents include nitrates and nitrites, benzoic acid, and calcium propionate.

ANTIOXIDANTS (oxygen interceptors, oxygen inhibitors, freshness preservers) slow the oxidation of oils and oil-based products. Oxidation, which causes food to turn rancid, occurs when oil is exposed to oxygen. Many vegetable oils contain the natural antioxidant, tocopherol (Vitamin E). Other natural antioxidants include ascorbic acid and citric acid. Most antioxidants in processed foods, however, are synthetic chemicals which destroy tocopherol. Many are toxic, and some may cause cancer. Antioxidants like BHA, BHT, and propyl gallate are used in many foods, including butter, cream, shortening, bacon, baked goods, powdered soup, fried food, margarine, candy, nuts, gelatin desserts, salad dressing, whipped topping, fruit drinks, breakfast bars, spices, peanut butter, bottled oil, canned fruits and vegetables, and foods which contain artificial color or flavor.

ANTISPLATTERING AGENTS like some of the silicones prevent oils from splattering when heated.

ANTISTALING AGENTS (antifirming agents, crumb-firming agents) such as glycerin keep baked goods from becoming stale by preventing the crystallization of starch. They are also used to improve the texture and volume of breads, cakes, doughnuts, etc.

BINDERS are starches and starchy products used to hold processed meats, snack foods, and other processed foods together. Many binders are natural substances like flour or bread crumbs which have been chemically treated to improve their binding ability.

BLEACHING AGENTS like benzoyl peroxide lighten the color of flour. Some only bleach while others also age the flour. (Also see maturing agents.) Bleaching agents can destroy Vitamin E and create a need for antioxidants. They are used in flour, bread, baked goods, as well as in some cheese, fats, and oils.

BREAD IMPROVERS are used to improve the consistency and handling properties of dough. (See animycotic agents, bleaching agents, dough conditioners, leaveners, maturing agents, and yeast foods.) Bread improvers are primarily used in breads and baked goods.

BUFFERS such as sodium acid pyrophosphate control the acidity and alkalinity of foods like soft drinks, cheese, chocolate products, cereals, syrups, baked goods, canned vegetables, jelly, dessert mixes, pasta, ham products, and ice cream. Buffers can hamper digestion and some can cause cavities.

CLARIFYING AGENTS (clarifiers, fining agents) are used to filter small particles out of liquids. Clarifying agents like egg white or tannin are used in the manufacture of vinegar, soft drinks, wine, beer, etc.

COLORS (food dyes, certified food colors, certified colors, FD&C lakes, FD&C colors) are natural or synthetic additives used to improve the appearance of processed foods like soft drinks, candy, ice cream, margarine, meat, meat products, butter, cheese, baked goods, gelatin desserts, pudding, icing, cereal, pasta, oranges, and maraschino cherries. More than 4 million pounds of colors are used each year, 95 percent of which are artificial. While artificial colors are now produced almost entirely synthetically, most were originally made from coal tar, a substance which causes cancer and other diseases even in small doses. Artificial colors are suspected of causing allergic reactions, hyperactivity among children, learning disorders, nerve tissue damage, and vision problems. A number of these nutritionless substances have already been banned, and the food industry is looking for safe, more nearly natural replacements for the few which are still approved. Colors now must be listed by name on food labels, but until recently only Yellow No. 5 (Tartrazine) had to be listed specifically. Colors are almost always used exclusively for cosmetic reasons.

CRYSTALLIZATION INHIBITORS (anticrystallization agents) such as iodine compounds prevent the formation of crystals which cloud oil and sugar products.

DOUGH CONDITIONERS make dough more easily managed and more controllable. Ammonium sulfate, benzoyl peroxide, and other chemicals are used to improve the processing and change the finished characteristics of bread, bread products, and other baked goods.

EMULSIFIERS (surface acting agents, surfactants, wetting agents) like polysorbates, mono- and diglycerides, lecithin, and propylene glycol help liquids like oil and water mix without separating. Although there are natural emulsifiers like eggs and milk, most are synthetic chemicals. They are found in most processed and convenience foods, including shortening, margarine, peanut butter, cakes and cake mixes, toppings, ice cream, soft drinks, some dairy products, processed meats, candy, pickles, nondairy creamer, chocolate, bread, and baked goods. Some emulsifiers, including some of the natural ones, may not be safe.

EXTENDERS and FILLERS are used to replace expensive ingredients with cheaper substitutes (like texturized vegetable protein) without reducing the volume or weight of the food. They are used in various processed foods, including lunch meats and other meat products.

FAT SUBSTITUTES are low-cholesterol, low-calorie replacements for fats in processed foods. Marketed under a variety of names, fat substitutes are used in a number of "designer" foods, such as low fat meats, frozen desserts, some fried foods, margarine, mayonnaise, dairy-type products, etc. Some, such as carrageenan, are forms of vegetable gum. Others may be made from egg or vegetable protein, grains, starches, fatty acids, carrageenan, or other sources. Many of the newer fat substitutes, such as sucrose polyester, have been produced in the laboratory and have no natural equivalents. Most are too new to have been tested thoroughly.

FIRMING AGENTS, including a number of salts, are used to preserve the texture and firmness of cut fruits and vegetables.

FLAVORS are the most common additives. More than 2,000 different flavors have been approved, most of which are complicated chemical compounds. They are used in most processed foods, usually in very small amounts, to replace or to supplement more expensive, real flavors. Few flavors, either natural or synthetic, have been tested, although many have been linked to allergic reactions, reproductive disorders, developmental problems, and other health disorders. Flavors must be described on labels by the words "natural," "real," or "artificial," but the actual chemicals used are seldom if ever listed. For information about specific chemicals used in flavors, see *A Consumer's Dictionary of Food Additives*, by Ruth Winter, which is listed in the bibliography.

FLAVOR CARRIERS such as brominated vegetable oil or propylene glycol are substances in which flavors are dissolved. The flavored carrier is then added to foods like soft drinks, syrups, candy, etc. Some flavor carriers may be dangerous.

FLAVOR ENHANCERS (flavor intensifiers, flavor potentiators, flavor modifiers) increase, accentuate, or modify the flavor of foods and sometimes improve the "mouthfeel" of processed foods. Substances like salt and MSG are added to soft drinks, ice cream, canned vegetables, soups and soup mixes, nondairy creamer, meat products, gelatin desserts, jelly, fruit drinks, sauces, gravies, etc. Some flavor enhancers (including IMP and GMP) are quite powerful, some (like MSG) can cause allergic reactions, and many others are up to sixty percent sodium, which has been associated with various health problems.

FOAMING AGENTS like sodium caseinate help foods foam or maintain foamy peaks.

HUMECTANTS (hydroscopic agents, water-retaining agents, moisture-retaining agents) like propylene glycol prevent foods from losing water and becoming brittle. They are used in moist foods like shredded coconut, icing, baked goods, chocolate, ice cream, candy, jelly, soft drinks, and diet food.

LEAVENERS (leavening agents) such as yeast or sodium bicarbonate release carbon dioxide into foods. This lightens the texture and makes preparation easier. Leaveners are used in baked goods, flour, cake mixes, brewed drinks, etc.

MATURING AGENTS like azodicarbonamide speed up the aging process of flour. Aging changes the protein in flour and allows the leaveners to make a fuller and more manageable dough. (See bleaching agents and leaveners.) Maturing agents are used in bread and baked goods.

NEUTRALIZERS (neutralizing agents) such as sodium carbonate act as preservatives by eliminating unwanted acidity in dairy products and other processed foods.

OLEORESINS are concentrated forms of flavor or color used in many processed foods. See solvents.

PRESERVATIVES keep food fresh and prolong shelf-life. (See acidifiers, antibrowning agents, antimycotic agents, antioxidants, antistaling agents, and sequestrants.) Not all preservatives are necessary, and some may be harmful. The food industry is exploring technological means of treating or packaging foods to replace these chemicals.

SEQUESTRANTS (chelators, chelating agents, sequestering agents) "tie up" or "bind" metallic ions which can contribute to deterioration, discoloration, and rancidity. Sequestrants like EDTA are used in fats, oils, beverages, and other foods which can suffer from oxidation. Because sequestrants bind metallic ions, they can also "lock up" trace elements which are useful for proper nutrition.

SOLVENTS are powerful chemicals used to make oleoresins. Herbs or spices can be steeped in a solvent to extract most of their available flavors. When the solvent is evaporated away, what remains is an oleoresin which can be used as a concentrated flavor or color. Solvents are also used for purposes like removing caffeine from coffee. Solvents are quite toxic, so it is important that they be totally evaporated out of the oleoresin.

STABILIZERS (stabilizing agents, suspending agents) such as gelatin make the texture and consistency of processed food uniform by preventing mixtures from separating or settling. They are often used with emulsifiers in foods like cocoa, baked goods, fruit drinks, puddings, and ice cream.

TEXTURIZERS like casein are used to improve the texture of canned goods, ice cream, frozen deserts, and other processed foods.

THICKENERS (bodying agents) thicken or improve the texture and consistency of various processed foods. Vegetable gums, cellulose, and other thickeners are used in puddings, soft drinks, salad dressing, soup, baby food, baby formula, ice cream, yogurt, jelly, etc.

YEAST FOODS like malt, sugar, calcium phosphate and other chemical salts nourish yeast and speed up the fermentation process. Yeast foods are found in foods which use or contain yeast, such as bread, baked goods, beer, and wine.

Chapter 6

Questionable Additives in Common Foods

Because modern food production depends heavily on standardized procedures, recipes, and techniques, similar foods are likely to contain similar additives. This makes careful shopping a little easier, because it allows the consumer to know that certain products are likely to contain certain additives. It is impossible to be totally sure, of course. A number of food manufacturers have responded to consumer pressure and removed at least some of the more controversial additives from their products. Nevertheless, it is useful to know that certain additives might be found in certain types of food.

This section lists specific categories of food and the questionable or suspicious additives they may contain. It is not a substitute for reading labels carefully. It lists only *selected* additives about which questions have been raised, not all the additives likely to be found in the product. And it makes generalizations which may not accurately describe specific food products. It is included as a general map to help you navigate your way through grocery-store aisles. Be sure to supplement the information here with the more detailed descriptions in the dictionary section of this guide.

BABY FOOD

carrageenan
modified starch
salt
sweeteners

CAKES, COOKIES, AND PASTRIES

BHA
BHT
artificial colors
artificial flavors
modified starch
salt
sulfites
sweeteners

CANNED FRUITS AND VEGETABLES

artificial colors
calcium salts
EDTA
salt
sulfites
sweeteners

CEREALS

artificial colors
artificial flavors
BHA
BHT
propyl gallate
salt
sweeteners

CONDIMENTS

benzoates
artificial colors
EDTA
GMP
IMP
modified starch
MSG
polysorbates
salt
sulfites
sweeteners

DAIRY PRODUCTS

carboxymethylcellulose
carrageenan
artificial colors
artificial flavors
GMP
hydrolyzed vegetable protein
IMP
MSG
phosphates
salt
sweeteners
vegetable gums

FLOUR PRODUCTS AND BAKED GOODS

artificial flavors
chlorine
corn syrup
dextrin
hydroxylated lecithin
modified starch
propionates

FLOUR PRODUCTS AND BAKED GOODS (continued)

salt
sulfites
sweeteners

FROZEN DESSERTS

artificial colors
artificial flavors
carrageenan
salt
sweeteners
vegetable gums

JAM AND JELLY

agar-agar
artificial colors
artificial flavors
benzoates
carboxymethylcellulose
carrageenan
propionates
sweeteners
solvents
vegetable gum

OILS, SPREADS, AND SHORTENING

artificial colors
artificial flavors
BHA
BHT
dimethylpolysiloxane
EDTA

OILS, SPREADS, AND SHORTENING (continued)

polysorbates
propyl gallate
salt

PASTA

disodium phosphate
salt
sulfites

PIES AND PIE FILLINGS

BHA
BHT
artificial colors
artificial flavors
modified starch
salt
sweeteners

POWDERED MIXES

artificial colors
artificial flavors
DSS
hydrolyzed vegetable protein
salt
sweeteners
vegetable gums

PREPARED AND CONVENIENCE FOODS

artificial colors
artificial flavors
carrageenan

PREPARED AND CONVENIENCE FOODS (continued)

GMP
hydrolyzed vegetable protein
IMP
modified starch
MSG
phosphates
salt
sweeteners
vegetable gums

PROCESSED MEATS AND MEAT PRODUCTS

artificial colors
artificial flavors
BHA
BHT
MSG
nitrates and nitrites
phosphates
propyl gallate
salt
sweeteners

PUDDING AND GELATIN DESSERTS

artificial colors
artificial flavors
BHA
carrageenan
polysorbates
salt
sweeteners

SALAD DRESSINGS AND MAYONNAISE

artificial colors
artificial flavors
BHA
BHT
carboxymethylcellulose
EDTA
GMP
IMP
modified starch
salt
sweeteners
vegetable gums

SAUCES AND GRAVIES

benzoates
hydrolyzed vegetable protein
salt
sweeteners
texturized vegetable protein

SNACK AND "JUNK" FOODS

artificial colors
artificial flavors
BHA
BHT
brominated vegetable oil
caffeine
GMP
hydrolyzed vegetable protein
IMP
modified starch
propyl gallate
salt
sulfites
sweeteners

SOUPS AND SOUP MIXES

artificial colors
artificial flavors
BHA
BHT
GMP
hydrolyzed vegetable protein
IMP
modified starch
MSG
propyl gallate
salt
sulfites
texturized vegetable protein

SOFT DRINKS

artificial colors
artificial flavors
caffeine
phosphoric acid
sweeteners

TOPPINGS AND ICINGS

artificial colors
artificial flavors
carrageenan
modified starch
polysorbates
sweeteners
vegetable gum

YOGURT

agar-agar
artificial colors
artificial flavors
carrageenan
gelatin
modified starch
pectin
sweeteners
vegetable gum

Chapter 7

A Dictionary of Common Additives

The most commonly used additives are described below in alphabetical order. At the minimum, each entry includes a description of how an additive is used and a partial list of the types of food it is used in. Within any description, an additive marked with an asterisk (*) is described in its own entry elsewhere in the dictionary.

Italicized additives are considered "Generally Recognized as Safe" by the FDA. (Bear in mind, however, that calling an additive safe does not make it safe. See the discussion of GRAS additives in Chapter 1, *Intentional Additives*, pages 11-12.) Every attempt has been made to ensure that the safety information presented below is accurate and up to date. However, the available information about additives is often changing and frequently contradictory. Even though the information has been carefully evaluated, there can be no guarantee that all inaccuracies have been eliminated. The simple fact that an additive is not called harmful does not mean that it is safe. Likewise, the association of a specific safety concern with an additive does not necessarily mean that it is dangerous.

Additives which may be associated with allergic reactions are followed by a black dot (•). Allergies are caused when proteins stimulate an immune system response. Among the more common sources of allergens are **corn, wheat, soy, nuts, peanuts, milk,** and **eggs.** But almost any protein can cause allergic reactions in sensitive individuals. An additive may cause an allergic reaction by itself. Or, it may be made from a substance which is allergenic. There is no absolute evidence that an additive made from an allergenic substance will necessarily cause an allergic reaction. On the other hand, there is also no evidence that the source of an additive is irrelevant to consumers with food allergies. Once again, consumers need to pay attention to their own personal reactions to foods which contain specific additives.

Acacia gum•   See gum Arabic, vegetable gums.

Acesulfame-K   See acesulfame potassium.

Acesulfame-potassium (acesulfame-K)   Artificial sweetener permitted in dry form and in dry mixes, gum, nondairy creamer, etc. Approval being sought for inclusion in baked goods and candies. May have caused breast and lung cancer and elevated cholesterol levels among lab animals. Marketed under name "Sunette." See sweeteners.

Acetic acid   Acidifier and occasional flavoring agent in candy, sauces, dressings, etc. Occurs naturally in vinegar; made synthetically from alcohol and acetaldehyde.

Acetone peroxide   Bleaching and maturing agent in flour. Used in small amounts in breads and other products made from processed flour. Often used with benzoyl peroxide*. Not thoroughly tested.

Acetylated mono- and diglycerides•   Emulsifier in candies. See mono- and diglycerides.

Adiptic acid   Acidifier in bottled drinks and occasionally in powdered drink mixes, gelatin desserts, etc.; occasionally preservative in oils.

Agar-agar•   Seaweed extract used as thickener, crystallization inhibitor, humectant, or stabilizer in soft drinks, ice cream, custard, ices, meringue, baked goods, jelly, icing, etc. Can act as laxative and cause allergic reactions.

Alginates (ammonium, potassium, sodium alginate; propylene glycol alginate)   Made from algin, a substance found in brown algae. Used as thickeners, stabilizers, foaming agent or crystallization inhibitors in foods including pastries, jelly, ice cream, cheese, yogurt, frosting, salad dressing, soft drinks, wine, beer, chocolate milk, and other prepared foods.

Alginic acid   Stabilizer or antifoaming agent in frozen desserts, cheese products, icings, salad dressings, and other processed foods. May be associated with birth defects and fetal deaths. See alginates.

Alpha tocopherol•   See tocopherol.

Alum   See aluminum sulfate.

Aluminum   Third most common element on earth's surface. Often occurs naturally in produce because of concentration in soil. Aluminum compounds used as anticaking agents, firming agents, alkalis, leaveners, etc. in baking powder, self-rising flour, cake mixes and pancake mixes, processed cheese, nondairy creamers, powders, etc. Also used in antacids and buffered aspirin as well as in cans, cartons and other packaging. Inadequately tested. Though poorly absorbed, has been ambiguously associated with senility and dementia-type diseases like Alzheimer's, Parkinson's, and amyotrophic lateral sclerosis (Lou Gehrig's Disease) and with kidney problems, neurological and memory problems, and mineral absorption deficiencies. Can concentrate in brain.

Aluminum ammonium sulfate Anticaking agent in salt and powders. See aluminum, ammonium.

Aluminum calcium silicate Anticaking agent in salt and powders. See aluminum, calcium, silicon.

Aluminum hydroxide Alkali or leavener in baked goods. See aluminum.

Aluminum potassium sulfate Anticaking agent or texturizer in pickles, cereal, flour, cheese, etc. See aluminum, potassium.

Aluminum sodium sulfate Used like aluminum potassium sulfate.

Aluminum sulfate (alum) Firming agent in pickles; used in manufacture of modified starch. See aluminum.

Ammonium Used in form of ammonium salt in variety of foods. May aggravate kidney and liver problems.

Ammonium alginate Stabilizer and humectant. See alginates, ammonium.

Ammonium bicarbonate Used instead of sodium bicarbonate* as alkali or leavener in some crackers and baked goods. See ammonium.

Ammonium carbonate Used like ammonium bicarbonate*.

Ammonium caseinate• Texturizer. See ammonium, casein.

Ammonium chloride Yeast food or dough conditioner in bread and baked goods. See ammonium.

Ammonium citrate Sequestrant, flavor enhancer, or firming agent. Salt of citric acid*. See ammonium.

Ammonium glutamate See ammonium, glutamates.

Ammonium hydroxide Alkali used like ammonium bicarbonate*. See ammonium.

Ammonium phosphate (monobasic and dibasic) Yeast foods, buffers, dough conditioners in bread and ingredients. Monobasic often used with sodium bicarbonate* in baking powder. See ammonium, phosphates.

Ammonium sulfate Yeast food, dough conditioner, or buffer in bread and baked goods. Used like ammonium phosphate*. See ammonium.

Ammonium sulfite• Preservative, antioxidant and antibrowing agent. See sulfites.

Amylases• Animal or vegetable enzymes which convert starch to sugar. Used as dough conditioners and bread improvers. Some may be made from soy.

Arabinogalactan• See larch gum, vegetable gums.

Artificial colors See section on colors in Chapter 2, *How Additives Are Used*, page 45.

Artificial flavors See section on flavors in Chapter 2, *How Additives Are Used*, page 46.

Artificial sweeteners See acesulfame-potassium, aspartame, cyclamates, and saccharin; also see sweeteners.

Ascorbates• Antioxidants in milk products, meat products, etc. Can affect mineral absorption. May provide source of Vitamin C and may prevent formation of nitrosamines (see nitrates and nitrites). Related to ascorbic acid*.

Ascorbic acid• (Vitamin C) Natural or synthetic vitamin supplement, acidifier, or antioxidant in soft drinks, cereals, processed meat, baked goods, frozen fruit, fruit juices, beer, candy, frozen desserts, etc. May be extracted from corn.

Ascorbyl palmitate Antioxidant or Vitamin C supplement in oils, fatty foods, candy, fortified foods, meat, canned fruit, etc. Related to ascorbic acid*.

Aspartame Artificial sweetener made from synthesis of two amino acids, phenylalanine and aspartic acid, with methanol (wood alcohol). Used in unheated diet foods, diet soft drinks, and powdered sugar substitutes. Can cause brain damage and retardation among phenylketonurics, who cannot process phenylalanine; may also cause brain chemistry changes, tumors, behavior change, headache, depression, seizures, hives, vision problems, menstrual difficulties, etc.; may also affect fetal brain development. Marketed as "Nutrisweet" or "Equal." See sweeteners.

Azodicarbonamide Maturing agent in flour. Often used with benzoyl peroxide*.

Baking powder• Dough conditioner used to replace yeast. Generally made from sodium bicarbonate* (baking soda), a starch, and an acid. May contain cornstarch*.

Benzoate of soda• (sodium benzoate) See benzoates, sodium.

Benzoates• Preservatives and antimycotic agents in pickles, salad dressing, fruit juice, soft drinks, jelly, margarine, mince meat, ice cream, baked goods, etc. Associated with allergic reactions, behavioral changes, water retention, intestinal upset, and perhaps hyperactivity in children. Should be avoided by people with liver problems.

Benzoic acid• Preservative and antimycotic agent. See benzoates.

Benzoyl peroxide Bleaching agent and dough conditioner in flour, oil, fat, and some milk products. Destroys Vitamin A and E; promotes oxidation and may increase concentration of oxidized fats.

Beta-carotene See carotene.

BHA• and *BHT•* (butylated hydroxyanisole and butylated hydroxytoluene) Antioxidants in oil, "junk food," potato chips, candy, gelatin desserts, margarine, baked goods, powdered soup, converted rice, soft drinks, sausages, cereal, chewing gum, shortening, packaging material, etc. Accumulate in body fat. Associated with kidney damage, allergies, behavioral changes, nerve and reproductive and immune system damage (both) and birth defects, cancer, and other organ damage (BHT). Should be avoided by infants, young children, and people sensitive to aspirin.

Brominated vegetable oil• Combination of bromine and vegetable oil. Used as flavor carrier or emulsifier in soft drinks, ice cream, baked goods, etc. Accumulates in body; linked to heart, liver, kidney, thyroid, spleen, pancreas, testicle damage, birth defects, and growth problems. May be based on corn, soy, or peanut oil. Removed from GRAS list in 1970.

1,3 butylene glycol Humectant or flavor carrier in flavored or color foods. May cause depression, drowsiness, and disorders of nervous, digestive, kidney, or respiratory systems.

Butylated hydroxyanisole• See BHA and BHT.

Butylated hydroxytoluene• See BHA and BHT.

Butylparaben Preservative, antimycotic agent related to benzoates*. See parabens.

BVO• See brominated vegetable oil.

Caffeine Common name of any of the *xanthine* family of natural stimulants. Found in tea, coffee, cocoa, kola beans, chocolate, used as flavoring agent in soft drinks, etc. Inconclusively associated with variety of health disorders, including high blood pressure, central nervous system stimulation, behavioral changes, birth defects, miscarriages, reduced fertility, heart problems, anxiety, insomnia, ulcer aggravation, osteoporosis, asthmatic reactions, etc. Can cross placental barrier to affect fetuses. May be associated with fibro-cystic breast lumps.

Calcium Compounds made from calcium. Probably safe and may be nutritionally useful. See specific calcium additives.

Calcium acetate Sequestrant. See acetic acid, calcium.

Calcium alginate Texturizer or gel. See alginates, calcium.

Calcium ascorbate• Antioxidant in milk products, processed meats, pickling brine, etc. Made from ascorbic acid* and calcium carbonate*. See also ascorbates, calcium.

Calcium bromate Occasionally used instead of potassium bromate* as maturing agent in flour, baked goods, etc. See calcium.

Calcium carbonate Yeast food, alkali, neutralizer, or flavor carrier in bread, wine, ice cream, syrup, candy, baking powder, etc. May cause constipation. See calcium.

Calcium caseinate• Texturizer made from surplus milk. See calcium, casein.

Calcium chloride Firming agent in canned fruit, canned tomatoes, jelly, pie filing, cheese, milk products, etc. See calcium.

Calcium citrate• Buffer in sweetened foods and saccharin and dough improver in baked goods. May be made from corn. See calcium, citric acid.

Calcium cyclamate See cyclamates, sweeteners.

Calcium disodium EDTA• Sequestrant and antioxidant. Can bind minerals. See EDTA.

Calcium fumarate• Acidifier of calcium* and fumaric acid*. May be made partially from corn.

Calcium gluconate• Calcium salt of gluconic acid* used as flavor enhancer, sequestrant, buffer, or firming agent in candy, confections, canned fruit and vegetables, soft drinks, etc. Made from sugar, possibly from corn sugar. See calcium.

Calcium hexametaphosphate Sequestrant, texturizer, or emulsifier in cereal, ice cream, milk products, beer, cake mixes, canned fish, pudding, diet jelly, etc. See calcium, phosphates.

Calcium hydroxide Firming agent in canned fruit. See calcium.

Calcium iodate Crystallization inhibitor or dough conditioner. See calcium, iodines.

Calcium lactate• Calcium salt of lactic acid* used as antibrowning agent or firming agent in fruits and vegetables, as yeast food in bread, and as buffer in soft drinks. Also used in evaporated milk. May be made from corn or milk. Also see calcium.

Calcium oxide (quicklime) Yeast food, dough conditioner, or alkali in bread, baked goods, dairy products, ice cream, sour cream, butter, candy, etc. See calcium.

Calcium peroxide Bleaching agent in bread and flour. See calcium.

Calcium phosphate (including monobasic calcium phosphate, dibasic calcium phosphate, and tribasic calcium phosphate) Bleaching agents, yeast foods, dough conditioners, or texturizers in flour and baked goods; often used with benzoyl peroxide*; monobasic also used in baking powder; tribasic also used as anticaking agent in salt, seasoned salt, vanilla powder, and other powders. See calcium, phosphates.

Calcium propionate• Antimycotic agent used in baked goods, chocolates, diet jellies, etc. May cause behavioral changes in small number of people. See calcium, propionates.

Calcium silicate Anticaking agent in baking powder and table salt. See calcium, silicons.

Calcium sodium EDTA• Sequestrant and antioxidant used like EDTA*. Linked to stomach upset and kidney damage; can also inhibit mineral use.

Calcium sorbate Preservative and antimycotic agent related to sorbic acid*.

Calcium stearate Anticaking agent in powdered foods. May be made from corn, peanuts, or soy. See calcium, stearic acid.

Calcium stearoyl-2-lactylate• Emulsifier, stabilizer, dough conditioner in baked goods and yeasted mixes. See stearoyls.

Calcium sulfate (plaster of Paris) Maturing agent, yeast food, dough conditioner, or alkali in flour, bread, brewed drinks, sherry, jelly, cereal, cheese, diet food, cottage cheese, etc. In flour, often used with benzoyl peroxide*. Can cause constipation.

Caprenin A fat substitute blended from fatty acids and designed for use in foods like candy bars. See "Fat Substitutes" in Chapter 5, *How Additives Are Used*, page 46.

Carboxymethylcellulose Modified form of cellulose, the basic ingredient in plant cells. Used (like other cellulose derivatives) as crystallization inhibitor, anticaking agents, texturizer, thickener, stabilizer, emulsifier, or humectant in ice cream, icing, candy, beer, jelly, pie filling, bread, pie crust, cake batter, diet drinks, salad dressing, soft drinks, whipped cream, syrup, processed cheese, etc. Made from wood or cotton which has been reacted with vinegar. May have caused cancer when injected under skins of rats.

Carob bean gum• See locust bean gum.

Carbon dioxide Gas used as propellant in pressurized cans and as source of carbonation in beverages.

Carotene Color and vitamin source in dairy products, margarine, shortening, etc.

Carrageenan Gel made from Irish Moss, a sea weed. Used as stabilizer, emulsifier, thickener, fat substitute, or crystallization inhibitor in milk products, chocolate products, frozen desserts, beer, infant formula, instant breakfast, dressing, baby food, whipped topping, ice cream, sour cream, jelly, syrup, and some pudding or gelatin desserts. May cause ulcers, particularly in infants; also associated with colitis and colon cancer.

Casein• Milk protein used as texturizer in frozen desserts and occasionally as cosmetic additive in "nondairy" creamer. Can cause allergic reactions among those sensitive to milk.

Cellulose gum See Carboxymethylcellulose.

Chlorine Bleaching and maturing agent in flour. Destroys Vitamin E. Chlorine can be incorporated into flour.

Chlorine dioxide Bleaching and maturing agent in flour. See chlorine.

Citric acid• Natural or synthetic acidifier, antioxidant or sequestrant in frozen desserts, canned meat, soft drinks, margarine, fruit juice, jelly, canned fruits and vegetables, cheese, candy, mayonnaise, instant potatoes, wine, salad dressing, crackers, etc. Can destroy tooth enamel and cause cavities. May be made from corn.

CMC See carboxymethylcellulose.

Colors See discussion in Chapter 2, *How Additives Are Used*, page 45.

Cornstarch• See starch.

Corn syrup• Made from corn or corn starch and used as sweetener, thickener, crystallization inhibitor, or humectant in a variety of processed foods. May be allergenic. See sweeteners.

Corn syrup solids• Dried corn syrup* for use in powdered foods like nondairy creamer. See sweeteners.

Cream of tartar See potassium acid tartrate.

Cuprous iodide Crystallization inhibitor and dough improver. See iodine.

Cyclamates Banned since 1969 as artificial sweeteners. Associated with mutations, testicular atrophy, and bladder cancer. See sweeteners.

*D**extrin*• Crystallization inhibitor, thickener, or antifoaming agent in milk, milk products, candy, beer, etc. Flavor carrier for oils in powdered foods. Made from starch of grains or cereals, including corn and wheat.

Dextrose• See glucose.

Diacetyl tartaric acid esters of mono- and diglycerides• Emulsifiers in shortening, bread, baked goods, etc. Related to mono- and diglycerides*.

Dibasic calcium phosphate See calcium phosphate.

Dibasic potassium phosphate See potassium phosphate.

Diglycerides• See mono- and diglycerides.

Dimethylpolysiloxane (methyl silicone, methyl polysilicone) A silicone* used as antifoaming or antisplattering agent in wine, syrup, sugar products, soft drinks, gelatin, soup, oil, etc. See silicon.

Dilauryl thiodipropionate Antioxidant in fats and oils.

Dioctyl sodium sulfosuccinate See DSS.

Dipotassium phosphate Sequestrant or buffer in cheese and non-dairy creamer.

Disodium EDTA• Sequestrant and antioxidant. See EDTA.

Disodium guanylate• Flavor enhancer. See GMP.

Disodium inosinate• Flavor enhancer. See IMP.

Disodium phosphate Sequestrant, emulsifier, binder, or buffer in evaporated milk, some cheeses, pasta, cured meat, soft drinks, sauces, chocolate products, beverages, toppings, etc. See sodium.

DSS (dioctyl sodium sulfosuccinate) Stabilizer or emulsifier in soft drinks, salad dressing, cocoa drinks, frozen desserts, etc. Also used as laxative. Not thoroughly tested; may have caused birth defects in large doses.

*E**DTA*• (ethylenediamine tetraacetic acid) Sequestrant and antioxidant in salad dressing, sandwich spreads, mayonnaise, margarine, seafood, canned goods, beer, soft drinks, etc. Linked to skin irritations, allergic reactions, liver and kidney damage, cramps, and mineral deficiencies.

Erythorbic acid• Antioxidant in pickles, meat, beverages, baked goods, etc. May be made from corn.

Ethoxylated mono- and diglycerides• Dough conditioners in yeasted baked goods. Not thoroughly tested. See mono- and diglycerides.

Ethyl cellulose   Binder or filler in candies, gum, and vitamins. See Carboxymethylcellulose.

Ethyl formate   Antimycotic agent in dried fruits, nuts, cereals, etc.; also used as flavoring agent. Occurs naturally in apples and coffee; also used in synthetic form.

Ethyl maltol•   Flavor enhancer five times stronger than the maltol* from which it is made. Used like maltol* and to hide the bitterness of saccharin*. May be made from corn or wheat.

Ethyl vanillin   Artificial vanilla* flavor. Associated with skin irritations, damage to reproductive and other organs, and cancer in lab animals.

Ethylenediamine tetraacetic acid•   See EDTA.

Fat substitutes (Caprenin, Olestra, Simplesse, Stellar, sucrose polyester) See "Fat Substitutes" in Chapter 5, *How Additives Are Used*, page 46.

Ferrous gluconate   Iron salt of gluconic acid*. Used like calcium gluconate* as flavor enhancer, sequestrant, buffer, or firming agent. Also used as coloring agent in black olives.

Flavors   See discussion in Chapter 5, *How Additives Are Used*, page 46.

Fructose• (levulose)   So-called natural or fruit sugar, actually more highly processed than sucrose and often has no connection to fruit. Mostly processed from cane or beet sugar or from corn. See sweeteners.

Fumaric Acid•   Acidifier in gelatin desserts, jelly, pudding, powdered soft drinks, candy, etc. Often combined with DSS* to improve ability to dissolve in water. May be made from corn.

Furcelleran•   Vegetable gum* made from seaweed. Used as emulsifier, stabilizer, or thickener in jellies, milk-based puddings, etc. Not adequately tested.

Gelatin Thickener, stabilizer, or crystallization inhibitor made from animal protein. Used in gelatin desserts, yogurt, frozen desserts, cheese spreads, some soft drinks, etc.

Gluconates•   Additives made from glucose* or gluconic acid*. See calcium, ferrous, potassium, and sodium gluconate.

Gluconic acid•   Acid made from glucose*. Used largely as part of other additives (gluconates*). May be derived from corn.

Glucono delta-lactone• Acidifier or leavener in baked goods, dairy products, processed fruit, juices, cured meats, etc. Made from glucose*, possibly derived from corn.

Glucose• Made from fruit, honey, sugar, or corn and used as sweetener or thickener in breads, soft drinks, syrups, some processed meats, etc. See sweeteners.

Glutamates• Flavor enhancers in meats and other processed foods based on amino acid, glutamate. Associated with brain and learning disorders, visual and behavioral problems, allergic reactions, etc. Pregnant women and young children should avoid. May be made from corn, soy, or wheat. See additional discussion under MSG.

Glutamic acid• Salt substitute and flavor enhancer in meats, beer, etc. See glutamates.

Glycerin• (glycerol) Humectant, flavor and color solvent, or antistaling agent in gelatin desserts, baked goods, candy, soft drinks, some meat products, etc. May be made from corn, peanuts, or soy.

GMP• (disodium guanylate, guanosine monophosphate) Powerful flavor enhancer often used with IMP* and MSG* in powdered soup, spreads, sauces, some canned vegetables, etc. Can be harmful to those with gout and similar diseases. Not thoroughly tested. May be made from soy or yeast.

Guar gum• Vegetable gum* made from guar plant. Stabilizer or thickener in soft drinks, ice cream, pudding, salad dressing, frozen fruit, fruit drinks, artificial toppings, processed meats, baked goods, cheese spreads, etc.

Gum Arabic• (acacia gum) Vegetable gum* made from acacia tree. Stabilizer or emulsifier in candy, jelly, beer, salad dressing, soft drinks, ice cream, glazes, chewing gum, etc. Also used as crystallization inhibitor. May cause allergic reactions and skin rashes; inadequately studied.

Gum ghatti• Vegetable gum* made from tree that grows in India. Stabilizer or emulsifier in syrup, salad dressing, soft drinks, etc. Also used as antifoaming agent. May be allergenic; not thoroughly tested.

Gum guaiac• Vegetable gum* made from guaiacum tree. Occasionally used as antioxidant in oils and fats.

Gum karaya• Vegetable gum* made from sterculia tree. Emulsifier or texturizer in gelatin products, whipped foods, salad dressing, sausages, ice cream, etc.; also used in commercial laxatives and cosmetics. Linked to allergies; not thoroughly tested.

Gum tragacanth• Vegetable gum* made from tree that grows in Iran. Thickener or stabilizer in salad dressing, frozen desserts, icings, jelly, and other acidic foods. May be allergenic; not thoroughly tested.

Heptylparaben• Preservative or antimycotic related to benzoates*. May cause birth defects in large doses. See parabens.

High-fructose corn syrup• Corn syrup* which has been treated with enzymes to make it sweeter. See sweeteners.

HPP• See hydrolyzed vegetable protein.

HVP• See hydrolyzed vegetable protein.

Hydrogen peroxide Bleaching agent, dough conditioner, or antimycotic agent in manufacture of baked goods, butter, cheese, etc. Also used to modify starch and to sterilize milk.

Hydrogenated vegetable oil• Polyunsaturated oil to which hydrogen has been added to keep the oil solid at higher temperatures, to prolong shelf-life, or to achieve certain baking or cooking qualities. Hydrogenated oils resemble saturated fats. Used in margarine, cooking oil, shortening, baked and fried foods, imitation milk, coffee creamer, peanut butter, etc. Has been associated with heart disease, hardening of arteries, and elevated cholesterol levels. May be based on corn, peanut, or soy oil.

Hydrolyzed plant protein• See hydrolyzed vegetable protein.

Hydrolyzed vegetable protein• Filler or flavor enhancer made from vegetable (usually soy) protein which has been broken by chemicals or enzymes to become water-soluble. Used in instant soup, canned meat dishes, hot dogs, gravy mixes, instant sauces, imitation meats, etc. May contain significant amounts of sodium*, MSG*, and glutamates*; may cause brain damage in infants, perhaps because of MSG; labels may no longer refer to HVP simply as "flavoring";may be made from corn, soy, or wheat protein.

Hydroxylated lecithin• Combination of lecithin* and peroxide. Used as antioxidant or emulsifier in ice cream, baked goods, margarine, etc. Not thoroughly tested.

Hydroxypropyl cellulose See carboxymethylcellulose.

Hydroxypropyl methylcellulose See carboxymethylcellulose.

IMP• (disodium inosinate, inosine monophosphate) Powerful flavor enhancer often used with GMP* and MSG*. May be made from soy or yeast. Similar in effects to GMP*.

Invert sugar• Made from glucose* and fructose*. Sweeter than table sugar. Used in candy and baked goods. See sweeteners.

Iodine Compounds made from iodine, a "trace element" necessary for proper thyroid functioning. Used as crystallization inhibitors in salt and as dough improvers in bread. Can cause goiter and thyroid disorders; may cause allergic-type reactions.

Irradiation Classified as additive by FDA. See discussion in Chapter 2, *Incidental Additives*, pages 26-7.

Isoascorbic acid• Antioxidant. See erythorbic acid.

Isolated soy protein• See soy isolates.

Isopropyl citrate• Antioxidant, sequestrant, acidifier made from citric acid*. Used in vegetable oils, margarine, and fatty foods.

*L**actic acid•*** Natural or synthetic acidifier, antioxidant, antimycotic agent, or buffer in bread, olives, cheese, baked goods, butter, beverages, beer, frozen desserts, etc. May be made from corn or milk.

Lactose• Milk sugar. Used in whipped toppings and some baked goods. Undigestible for some people. Can cause liver and eye problems and mental retardation among galactosemics who lack enzyme to digest; can also cause gas, bloating, diarrhea, etc. among intolerant adults.

Lactyllic Stearate• Dough conditioner in bread and baked goods. May cause allergic reactions. See stearic acid.

Larch gum • (arabinogalactan) Made from western larch tree. Occasionally used as stabilizer, emulsifier, binder, or thickener in artificial sweeteners, salad dressings, puddings, dry soup mixes, sauces, etc. May contain excessive amounts of tannin*. Not thoroughly tested.

Lecithin• Emulsifier, stabilizer, thickener, crystallization inhibitor, or antioxidant usually made from soybeans, corn, eggs, or peanuts but present in a number of foods. Used in cereal, margarine, oil products, chocolate, frozen desserts, soft drinks, baked goods, etc. May reduce cholesterol levels in arteries.

Levulose• See fructose.

Linoleic acid•   Fatty acid used as ingredient in emulsifiers and vitamins. May be made from soy, peanuts, or corn.

Locust bean gum•   (carob bean gum; Saint John's bread gum) Made from carob tree. Thickener, texturizer, stabilizer in ice cream, salad dressing, pie filling, barbecue sauce, whipped foods, cheese products, etc.; also used as dough improver in baked goods. May lower blood cholesterol.

Magnesium   Compounds made from magnesium and used as buffers, neutralizers, alkalies, or anticaking agents in soft drinks, baked goods, dairy products, cocoa, brewed drinks, canned vegetables, salt, seasoned salt, powders, etc. May be harmful for people with kidney problems; some can be toxic in large amounts.

Magnesium acetate   Buffer, neutralizer, alkali, or anticaking agent. See magnesium.

Magnesium carbonate   Alkali or anticaking agent in dairy products, chocolate products, canned vegetables, etc. Often used with benzoyl peroxide* as bleaching or maturing agent in flour, baked goods, etc. See magnesium.

Magnesium chloride   Firming agent or color preservative in canned vegetables. See magnesium.

Magnesium fumarate•   Acidifier of magnesium* and fumaric acid*. May be made partially from corn.

Magnesium hydroxide   Alkali in canned vegetables. See magnesium.

Magnesium oxide   Neutralizer in frozen foods, canned vegetables, butter, etc. See magnesium.

Magnesium silicate   Anticaking agent in salt and powders. See magnesium and silicon. May have caused kidney damage in dogs.

Malic acid•   "Apple acid." Natural or synthetic acidifier in fruit drinks, baked goods, candy, iced tea mix, butter, ice cream, dairy products, jelly, etc. May also be made from corn.

Maltodextrin•   Texturizer and flavor enhancer in candies. May be made from corn.

Maltol•   Flavor enhancer used in baked goods, gelatin desserts, ice cream, soft drinks, and other sweetened foods. May be made from corn or wheat.

Maltose•   Malt sugar used as sweetener and in diabetic food. May be made from corn, soy, or wheat.

Mannitol• Sugar "alcohol" used as sweetener or texturizer in gum, diet products, etc. Even in small amounts can cause diarrhea and gastric upset, particularly in infants, and act as both laxative and diuretic; can also cause or aggravate kidney disorders. May be made from sugar, seaweed, or corn.

Methyl polysilicone See methyl silicone, silicon.

Methylparaben• Preservative, antimycotic agent related to benzoates*. May have caused birth defects in lab animals. See parabens.

Methylcellulose Thickener or stabilizer in beverages, canned fruit, baked goods, etc. See Carboxymethylcellulose.

Methyl silicone (methyl polysilicone) Antifoaming or antisplattering agent in oils. See dimethylpolysiloxane, silicon.

Modified starch• Corn, wheat, or other starch subjected to chemicals or acids to modify physical or chemical characteristics and allow it to dissolve in liquids. Thickener, anticaking agent, or humectant in sugar, baking powder, pie filling, frozen food, baby food, etc. Some of the chemicals used to manufacture linked to heart, kidney, and intestinal disorders. Also see starch.

Mono- and diglycerides• (and additives made from them) Dough conditioners, antistaling agents, antifoaming agents, stabilizers, crystallization inhibitors, or emulsifiers in bread, baked goods, peanut butter, chocolate, whipped toppings, margarine, candy, frozen desserts, jelly, etc. Made from fats or corn, peanut, or soy oil.

Monobasic calcium phosphate See calcium phosphate.

Monobasic potassium phosphate See potassium phosphate.

Monoammonium glutamate• Flavor enhancer. See glutamates.

Monopotassium glutamate• Flavor enhancer. See glutamates.

Monosodium glutamate• (MSG) Sodium salt of glutamic acid*. Flavor enhancer in many processed foods, including soup and soup mixes, canned vegetables, bouillon, processed fish, frozen food, canned meat, seasonings, salad dressings, mayonnaise, baked goods, potato chips, etc. Allergic reactions ("Chinese Restaurant Syndrome") are common; caused brain lesions and eye damage in lab animals; may not be safe for human fetuses or infants; linked to reproductive disorders, fertility problems, learning disorders; reactions can mimic symptoms of heart attack. Should be avoided by nursing mothers and infants. No longer added directly to baby foods. Ingredients which may contain MSG must now be listed on labels. May be made from soy, sugar, seaweed, corn, or wheat. Also see glutamates.

Monosodium phosphate Emulsifier, buffer, or humectant in cereals, processed meats, etc.

Monosodium phosphate derivatives of mono- and diglycerides• Emulsifiers made from fats, oils, or fatty acids. See mono- and diglycerides.

MSG• See monosodium glutamate.

Nitrates and **nitrites** Antimycotic agents and colors in processed meats like bacon, hot dogs, lunch meat, canned or packaged ham, sausage, etc. Nitrites pose greater health risks, but nitrates can be converted to nitrites by digestive juices. Can be toxic in moderate amounts; linked to cancer, brain damage, arthritis, anemia, etc.; can turn into powerful carcinogens, nitrosamines and nitrosophyrroidine; considered dangerous by FDA but not banned because of ability to prevent botulism, especially in canned hams; should be avoided by infants.

Nitrosyl chloride Bleaching or maturing agent in flour, baked goods, etc.

Oat gum• Vegetable gum* used as antioxidant, thickener, or stabilizer in dairy products, candy, etc. Occasionally allergenic; may cause intestinal upset.

Oleic acid Antifoaming agent, flavor carrier, or binder in frozen desserts, baked goods, beverages, etc.

Olestra A fat substitute made from fatty acids chemically bonded to sugar molecules. Designed to be nondigestible and usable in fried foods. See "Fat Substitutes" in Chapter 5, *How Additives Are Used*, page 46.

Oxystearin Modified fatty acid used as crystallization inhibitor in mayonnaise, salad dressing, sugar, yeast, etc. Related to mono- and diglycerides*.

Papain• Enzyme from papaya plant. Used as meat tenderizer. May be allergenic; can aggravate ulcers; taken raw and in large amounts can interfere with digestion.

Parabens• (parahydroxybenzoic acid compounds) Very common preservatives or antimycotic agents related to benzoates*. Used in diet foods, fats, oils, frozen desserts, milk products, baked goods, jelly, etc. Not thoroughly tested; should be avoided by people sensitive to aspirin.

Partially hydrogenated vegetable oil See hydrogenated vegetable oil.

Pectin Natural gelling agent, thickener, stabilizer, or emulsifier in jelly, barbecue sauce, salad dressing, yogurt, cranberry sauce, frozen desserts, canned frosting, soft drinks, syrup, etc.

Phosphates Sequestrants, emulsifiers, acidifiers, or texturizers in evaporated milk, soft drinks, oil, baked goods, etc. Can interfere with absorption of calcium and other minerals; can cause kidney damage in large amounts. Related to phosphoric acid*. See phosphorus.

Phosphoric acid Acidifier in frozen desserts, soft drinks, jelly, some dairy products, baked goods, candy, cheese, and brewed drinks. Sequestrant in animal fats. Can destroy tooth enamel and interfere with calcium absorption. See phosphates.

Phosphorus Compounds made from phosphorus, usually phosphoric acid* or one of the phosphates*. Excess can lead to calcium deficiency, poor bone and tooth development, and possibly osteoporosis. Commonly found in cola and other soft drinks.

Polydextrose• Compound of dextrose*, sorbitol*, and citric acid*. Filler or sugar substitute in diet food, puddings, candy, frozen deserts, baked goods, etc. May act as laxative or cause gas. May be made from corn.

Polyoxyethylene sorbitan monooleate• (polysorbate 80) Emulsifier made from sorbitol* and oleic acid*. See polysorbates.

Polyoxyethylene sorbitan monostearate• (polysorbate 60) Emulsifier made from sorbitol* and stearic acid*. See polysorbates.

Polyoxyethylene sorbitan tristearate• (polysorbate 65) Emulsifier made from sorbitol* and stearic acid*. See polysorbates.

Polyoxyethylene stearate Texturizer and cosmetic additive used in baked goods. Made from stearic acid*.

Polysorbates• Compounds of polyoxyethylene sorbitan and fatty acids. Related to sorbitol*. Emulsifiers or antifoaming agents in gelatin products, salad dressings, baked goods, candy, soup, ice cream, nondairy creamer, artificial toppings, chocolate, pickles, spreads, soft drinks, etc. May be made from corn, peanuts, or soy.

Potassium Any of a number of compounds made from the element, potassium. Normally used as buffers, preservatives, or yeast foods in soft drinks, brewed drinks, diet jelly, candy, etc. Large amounts of potassium may be harmful to those with kidney or heart problems.

Potassium acid tartrate (cream of tartar) Leavener, anticaking agent, acidifying agent, etc. in baked goods, processed foods, carbonated beverages. See potassium, tartaric acid.

Potassium alginate Thickener or stabilizer. See potassium and alginates.

Potassium benzoate See benzoates, potassium.

Potassium bicarbonate Leavener in baked goods and "general purpose" additive. Occasionally used instead of sodium bicarbonate*. See potassium.

Potassium bisulfite• Antimycotic agent, preservative in brewed drinks and fruit products. See potassium, sulfites.

Potassium bromate Maturing agent used in flour and flour products. Has been linked to tumors, kidney failure, cancer, mutations, and possible central nervous system damage. Promotes oxidation of fats and oils.

Potassium carbonate Alkali in cocoa products and confections.

Potassium caseinate Texturizer made from surplus milk. Used as texturizer in frozen desserts. See casein, potassium.

Potassium chloride Yeast food, salt substitute, or buffer in brewed drinks, soft drinks jelly, and some baked goods. Linked to ulcers and digestive disorders; may aggravate heart, liver, and kidney problems.

Potassium citrate• Antioxidant, sequestrant, buffer, or acidifier made from potassium* and citric acid*.

Potassium fumarate• Acidifier of potassium* and fumaric acid*. May be made partially from corn.

Potassium gluconate• Potassium salt of gluconic acid*. Used like calcium gluconate* as flavor enhancer, sequestrant, buffer, or firming agent. Also used as buffer in carbonated water. May be made from corn. See potassium.

Potassium glutamate Flavor enhancer made from glutamic acid*· and potassium*. See glutamates.

Potassium iodate Anticaking agent and dough improver. See iodine and potassium.

Potassium iodide Anticaking agent, mineral supplement, and dough improver. See iodine and potassium.

Potassium metabisulfite• Preservative, antioxidant, and antibrowning agent. See sulfites, potassium.

Potassium nitrate Antimycotic agent and color preservative. See nitrates and nitrites.

Potassium nitrite Antimycotic agent and color preservative. See nitrates and nitrites.

Potassium phosphate (monobasic, dibasic, and tribasic) Yeast foods in brewed drinks. See phosphates, potassium.

Potassium sorbate Preservative, antimycotic agent in drinks, baked goods, syrups, fruit products, processed salads, desserts, diet jellies, etc. See potassium, sorbic acid.

Potassium sulfite• Preservative, antioxidant, and antibrowning agent. See sulfites, potassium.

Propionates• (propionic acid; calcium and sodium propionate) Antimycotic agents in bread, baked goods, stuffing, cheese, and chocolate. May cause allergic reactions and occasional behavioral changes.

Propionic acid• Preservative found naturally in Swiss cheese. See propionates.

Propyl gallate• Antioxidant often used with BHA* and BHT* in oil, meat products, soft drinks, ice cream, candy, nuts, dried soup, gelatin desserts, baked goods, chewing gum, etc. Linked to liver and kidney damage, cancer, lymphoma, reproductive problems, allergic reactions, etc.

Propylene glycol• Humectant, flavor carrier, or texturizer in chocolate, candy, toppings, soft drinks, baked goods, canned icing, meat products, coconut, etc. May cause allergic rash.

Propylene glycol alginate• Stabilizer and antifoaming agent in salad dressings and frozen desserts. See alginates, propylene glycol.

Propylene glycol monostearate• Emulsifier and dough conditioner in baked goods, oils, etc. May be made from corn, peanuts, or soy.

Propylparaben• Preservative, antimycotic agent related to benzoates*. See parabens.

*Q*uicklime See calcium oxide.

Quinine Natural flavor used in tonic water and bitter drink mixers. May cause miscarriages, deafness and hearing difficulties, rashes, and other reactions.

*R*ennet   Enzyme used to coagulate milk in cheese and some desserts. Usually extracted from stomachs of slaughtered calves; occasionally made from plant sources.

*S*accharin   Artificial sweetener used in diet foods and soft drinks. Linked to bladder cancer. GRAS until 1972. FDA has tried to ban since 1977. Warning label required. See sweeteners.
Saint John's bread gum•   See locust bean gum.
Salt   Technically, a chemical union of a metal and an acid. Commonly used as another name for sodium chloride*.
SAPP   See sodium acid pyrophosphate.
Silica   Anticaking agents. See silicon.
Silicates   Anticaking agents. See silicon.
Silicon dioxide   Anticaking agent. See silicon.
Silicones   Antifoaming or antisplattering agents. See silicon.
Silicon   Any of a number of additives made from the element, silicon, including:

> **Silica** (silicon dioxide) and **silicates**, which are anticaking agents in powdered foods like salt, nondairy creamer, dry soup mixes, vanilla powder, baking powder, etc.
> **Silicones** (like dimethylpolysiloxane), which are antifoaming or antisplattering agents in wines, syrup, soft drinks, sugar, gelatin, soup, vegetable oil, yeast, etc.

Some silicon additives, particularly those silicates which are combined with magnesium or sodium, may cause kidney problems. Asbestos contamination is possible in some silicates.
Simplesse   A fat substitute made from milk or egg proteins and designed for use in variety of processed foods, including frozen desserts, dairy-type products, mayonnaise, etc .See "Fat Substitutes" in Chapter 5, *How Additives Are Used*, page 46.
Sodium   A number of major additives are based on the element, sodium, including sodium chloride* (salt). It is largely the sodium which causes most of the problems people experience with salt and other sodium additives, including high blood pressure, water retention, kidney dysfunction, etc. Salt and sodium additives amount to about ten percent of all additives.
Sodium acetate   Buffer in soft drinks. Preservative in candy. See acetic acid, sodium.

Sodium acid pyrophosphate (SAPP) Buffer or leavener in prepared cakes, cake mixes, other baked goods, etc. Also used in curing processed meats like hot dogs, sausage, tuna, etc. See sodium, phosphates.

Sodium alginate Thickener, stabilizer, crystallization inhibitor. See alginates, sodium.

Sodium aluminum phosphate Used with sodium bicarbonate* in baking soda. Also used in cheese. See aluminum, sodium, phosphates.

Sodium aluminum sulfate Aluminum "salt" which forms the "SAS" in many baking powders. Used in products like baked goods which employ baking powder. Often used with benzoyl peroxide* as bleaching and maturing agent in flour. Has been associated with kidney failure in rats. See sodium, aluminum.

Sodium ascorbate• Antioxidant in meat products. See ascorbates, sodium.

Sodium benzoate• (benzoate of soda) Preservative and antimycotic agent. See benzoates, sodium.

Sodium bicarbonate (baking soda) Leavener in large number of baked goods. Also used as buffer in soft drinks, soups, frozen desserts, syrup. See sodium.

Sodium bisulfite• Antioxidant, antimycotic agent, or antibrowning agent. See sulfites, sodium.

Sodium calcium aluminosilicate Anticaking agent. See silicon.

Sodium carboxymethylcellulose See carboxymethylcellulose, sodium.

Sodium carbonate Neutralizer in butter, milk products, olives, cocoa products, etc. See sodium.

Sodium caseinate• Texturizer made from surplus milk. Used in frozen desserts, processed meats, and nondairy creamer. See casein, sodium.

Sodium chloride Flavor enhancer and occasional preservative in large number of processed foods. Consumed in excessive amounts by most people, largely from processed and "fast" food. Linked to high blood pressure, water retention, kidney disease. See sodium.

Sodium citrate Acidifier and antioxidant used like citric acid*. Also used as emulsifier, buffer, or sequestrant in some milk products, beverages, candies, jellies, etc. See sodium.

Sodium cyclamate See cyclamates, sweeteners.

Sodium diacetate Antimycotic agent in bread and baked goods.

Sodium erythorbate• (sodium isoascorbate) Antioxidant in processed meat, beverages, potato salad, baked goods, etc. Related to ascorbic acid* and ascorbates*. May be made from corn. See sodium.

Sodium ferrocyanide See yellow prussiate of soda.

Sodium fumarate• Acidifier made from sodium* and fumaric acid*. May be based partially on corn.

Sodium gluconate• Sodium salt of gluconic acid* used as sequestrant. Also see sodium.

Sodium hexametaphosphate Emulsifier, stabilizer, sequestrant, or thickener in soft drinks, cereal, baked goods, fish, ice cream, juice concentrate, pudding, cheese, jelly, etc. See sodium, phosphates.

Sodium hydroxide (caustic soda, soda lye) Alkali or neutralizer used in production of modified starch and in pretzels, vegetable oil, animal fat, sour cream, butter, cocoa products, canned vegetables, etc.

Sodium isoascorbate• See sodium erythorbate.

Sodium metabisulfite• Preservative, antimycotic agent, antibrowning agent. See sulfites, sodium.

Sodium metaphosphate Dough conditioner. See sodium hexametaphosphate.

Sodium nitrate Antimycotic agent and color preservative. See nitrates and nitrites, sodium.

Sodium nitrite Antimycotic agent and color preservative. See nitrates and nitrites, sodium.

Sodium pectinate Thickener or stabilizer in frozen desserts, candies, dressings, jellies, etc. See pectin, sodium.

Sodium potassium tartrate Emulsifier or acidifying agent in cheese, fats, jelly, etc. See sodium, potassium, tartaric acid.

Sodium propionate• Antimycotic agent in baked goods, etc. See sodium, propionates. Can contribute to salt-related problems.

Sodium pyrophosphate Thickener, emulsifier, sequestrant in canned meats, cheese, puddings, etc. See sodium, phosphates.

Sodium sesquicarbonate Neutralizer in milk products, olives, cocoa products, etc. See sodium.

Sodium silicate Anticaking agent. See sodium, silicon.

Sodium silicoaluminate Anticaking agent. See sodium, silicon, aluminum.

Sodium sorbate Antimycotic agent or antibrowning agent. See sodium, sorbic acid.

Sodium stearoyl fumarate• Dough conditioner, bread improver, or emulsifier in baked goods, whipped cream, frozen desserts, icing, filling, shortening, etc. See stearoyls.

Sodium stearoyl-2-lactylate• Emulsifier, stabilizer, or dough conditioner used like calcium stearyl-2-lactylate*. See stearoyls.

Sodium sulfate Buffer in soft drinks. See sodium.

Sodium sulfite• Antimycotic agent, antibrowning agent, or preservative in wine, distilled drinks, juices, syrups, processed fruits and vegetables, etc. See sodium, sulfites.

Sodium sulfoacetate mono- and diglycerides• Emulsifiers and antisplattering agents in margarine. Not thoroughly tested. See mono- and diglycerides.

Sodium tartrate Emulsifier, acidifying agent in cheese, fat, jelly, etc. See sodium, tartaric acid.

Sodium thiosulfate Antioxidant used in potato products.

Sodium tripolyphosphate (STPP) Texturizer or sequestrant in modified starch, canned meat, etc. See sodium, phosphates.

Sorbic acid Antimycotic or antibrowning agent in dried fruit, chocolate, baked goods, margarine, syrup, soft drinks, jelly, cheese, prepared salads, wine, canned frosting, etc.

Sorbitan monopalmitate• Emulsifier occasionally used in baked goods instead of sorbitan monostearate*. May be made from corn, peanuts, or soy.

Sorbitan monostearate• Emulsifier, stabilizer, or antifoaming agent in baked goods, oil-based icings and toppings, candies, etc. Often used with a polysorbate*. May be made from corn, peanuts, or soy.

Sorbitan tristearate• Emulsifier occasionally used in candies instead of sorbitan monostearate*. May be made from corn, peanuts, or soy.

Sorbitol• A sugar "alcohol" used in soft drinks, candy, coconut, diet food, etc. Can act as laxative and cause diarrhea and gastrointestinal problems, particularly among infants and young children. May be made from corn. See sweeteners.

Soy concentrates• Texturized and concentrated soy protein. Used with other additives and flavors as fillers or extenders in imitation meats. See soy isolates, texturized vegetable protein.

Soy isolates• Highly processed soy concentrates. Used as fillers in imitation meats and soy products like infant formula and iced desserts. May include numerous other additives.

Stannous chloride Antioxidant in soft drinks and canned vegetables.

Starch• Natural thickener made from corn, wheat, potatoes, etc. Used in soup, gravy, etc. Often combined with other chemicals to form modified starch*.

Stearic acid Fatty acid used in chewing gum and as basis for other additives.

Stearoyl propylene glycol hydrogen succinate• See succistearin.

Stearoyls• Dough conditioners, bread improvers, emulsifiers in baked goods, whipped cream, frozen desserts, icing, fillings, shortening, dehydrated foods, etc. May be made from corn, milk, peanuts, or soy.

Stearyl citrate• Antioxidant, sequestrant primarily used in margarine. Related to citric acid* and stearic acid*.

Stearyl-2-lactyllic acid Emulsifier in shortening, baked goods, cake mixes, icing, filling, etc.

Stellar See "Fat Substitutes" in Chapter 5, *How Additives Are Used*, page 46.

STPP See sodium tripolyphosphate.

Succinic acid Buffer, neutralizing agent, and ingredient in other additives. Made from acetic acid*.

Succistearin• (stearoyl propylene glycol hydrogen succinate) Emulsifier occasionally used in shortening used in baked goods. See propylene glycol, stearic acid.

Sucrose White and brown sugar. See sweeteners.

Sucrose polyester A fat substitute made from fatty acids chemically bonded to sugar molecules. Marketed under the name, *Olestra*. See "Fat Substitutes" in Chapter 5, *How Additives Are Used*, page 46.

Sulfites• Sulfur-based preservatives, antioxidants, and antibrowning agents in wine, sugar, molasses, fresh and dried fruit and vegetables, juices, seafood, pasta, condiments, "junk food," meats, etc. Can cause allergic reactions, asthma, and anaphylactic shock in small doses; dangerous for people suffering from asthma; destroy Vitamin B-1 (Thiamine). Sulfites have caused deaths among very sensitive people. Banned for use on fresh fruits and vegetables.

Sulfur dioxide• Preservative, antioxidant, antibrowning agent. See sulfites.

Sulfuric acid Acidifier, buffer, in brewed drinks; used to modify starch.

Sweeteners Sweetness is the seductive taste, which may explain why sweeteners are the most heavily used additives in processed foods. Most sweeteners take the form of refined (simple) sugar— white and brown sugar, maple sugar, maple syrup, corn sugar, corn syrup, molasses, honey, and other sugars ending in the suffix, *-ose*.

Very few nutritional differences exist among these refined sugars. Many are simply modified forms of white sugar. "Raw" or "turbinado" sugar is merely unbleached and slightly less processed white sugar. Molasses (which may contain sulfites*) is the liquid which remains after cane or beet sugar has been processed. Confectioner's sugar is finely pulverized white sugar to which cornstarch may have been added. Brown sugar is white sugar with molasses or molasses color added. Maple sugar and maple syrup are refined products of the sap of maple trees and may contain residues of harsh chemicals used to increase the sap flow. Honey, which may or may not be less processed than other sugars, is sweeter and stickier than sugar and may contribute more to tooth decay. Honey may also contain botulism spores (which are particularly hazardous for infants) or pesticide residues.

Sugar is a nutritional nightmare. Most sugar is consumed in soft drinks, "junk" food, breakfast cereals, and other foods which offer little nutritional value. Almost all sugars are associated with physical and emotional disorders, such as tooth decay, B-vitamin deficiency, hypoglycemia, diabetes, hyperactivity, fatigue, depression, and possibly immune system dysfunction. Some believe that sugar is addictive, psychologically at least. Finally, the overeating of both sugar and the highly processed "junk" foods which contain sugar is a major factor in the weight problems experienced by many people. The average American eats approximately 125 pounds of sugar annually. This is the equivalent of 227,000 calories, or approximately 65 pounds of body weight per year!

Particularly because of the association of sugar with both weight and blood-sugar disorders, a number of sugar substitutes have been developed. Some of these, such as the sugar alcohols (mannitol*, sorbitol*, xylitol*) are "natural," but few are free of health problems. Others are totally synthetic and potentially harmful. Cyclamates*, once the principle artificial sweeteners, were banned when they were linked to birth defect and cancer. Saccharin*, which replaced cyclamates, is also thought to cause cancer, kidney disease, and birth defects. FDA attempts to ban saccharin from use in food have been diverted by industry pressure and Congressional intervention. More recent sugar substitutes include aspartame* and acesulfame-potassium*, neither of which may be totally safe. Ironically for dieters, these sugar substitutes may actually encourage the overeating of sweets by reinforcing the taste for sweet foods.

*T**annic acid* (tannin)   Clarifying agent and flavor used in oils, wine, baked goods, butter, caramel, liquid flavorings, etc. Found naturally in coffee, tea, wine, etc. May cause cancer of liver or esophagus.
Tannin   See tannic acid.
Tartaric acid   Acid found in grapes. Used as acidifier in frozen desserts, soft drinks, baking powder, jelly, baked goods, candy, diet jelly, etc.
TBHQ (tertiary butylhydroquinone)   Antioxidant normally used with BHA and BHT. Can cause nausea in moderately large amounts; may cause behavioral problems among children; inadequately tested.
Tertiary butylhydroquinone   See TBHQ.
Texturized vegetable protein• (TVP)   Soy protein chemically treated, shaped, flavored, or colored to resemble other foods. Used as extender, filler, or replacement in imitation meats such as bacon bits, "soyburger," etc. Additives and chemicals used in processing may include salt, flavor enhancers, artificial colors and flavors, etc.
THBP (2-4-5 Trihydroxybutrophenone)   Antioxidant in oils and oil-based products.
Tocopherol• (Vitamin E)   Natural or synthetic antioxidant in fats, oils, and oil-based products. May be made from corn, peanuts, or soy.
Tribasic calcium phosphate   See calcium phosphate.
Tribasic potassium phosphate   See potassium phosphate.
Tricalcium silicate   Anticaking agent. See silicon.
2-4-5 Trihydroxybutrophenone   See THBP.
TVP   See texturized vegetable protein.

*V**anilla*   The most common food flavor. Natural vanilla, made from an orchid, is becoming rare, so the flavor has been approximated synthetically as vanillin* and ethyl vanillin*.
Vanillin   Synthetic vanilla flavor. See vanilla.
Vegetable gums•   Gum-like substances extracted from plants and parts of plants not normally eaten. Used mainly as thickeners, gels,

stabilizers, emulsifiers, binders, or humectants in variety of processed foods. Most can cause allergic reactions or act as laxatives; most are not thoroughly tested. See furcelleran, guar gum, gum Arabic, gum ghatti, gum guaiac, gum karaya, gum tragacanth, larch gum, locust bean gum, oat gum, and xanthan gum.

Veratraldehyde Flavor enhancer in soft drinks, ice cream, candy, baked goods, pudding, etc. Made from vanillin*.

Xanthan Gum• Made from corn syrup. Thickener, stabilizer, emulsifier in dairy products, salad dressing, baked goods, vegetable protein products, etc.

Xylitol Sugar alcohol made from birch wood. Used occasionally in chewing gum and tooth paste. Linked to cancer, bladder problems, diarrhea, liver problems, cramps. Some manufacturers refuse to use.

Yeast-malt sprout extract• Flavor enhancer in sauces, gravies, etc.

Yellow prussiate of soda (sodium ferrocyanide) Anticaking agent used in salt and powders.

Chapter 8
Other Selected Sources of Information

General Books About Foods and Food Safety

Michael F. Jacobson, Ph.D., Lisa Y. Lefferts, and Anne Witte Garland, *Safe Food: Eating Wisely in a Risky World* (Los Angeles: Center for Science in the Public Interest and Living Planet Press, 1991).

An excellent and comprehensive discussion of food safety issues. Jacobson is the Executive Director of the Center for Science in the Public Interest, one of the most active organizations in defense of consumer health and safety. Foreword by Ralph Nader. Recommended.

Christopher S. Kilham, *The Bread & Circus Whole Food Bible* Reading: Massachusetts: Addison-Wesley Publishing Company, Inc., 1991).

Another comprehensive guide, considerably more critical but still quite informative. Includes recipes.

John Tepper Marlin, Ph.D., with Domenick M. Bertelli, *The Catalogue of Healthy Food* (New York: Bantam Books, 1990).

An excellent introduction which also includes comprehensive information about shopping for healthy foods and lists of actions concerned consumers can take. Recommended.

Patrick Quillin, Ph.D., *Safe Eating* (New York: M. Evans and Company, Inc., 1990)

A wide-ranging discussion of food safety problems and consumer-oriented solutions. Includes several relevant topics not discussed in other books on food safety. Useful.

David Steinman, *Diet for a Poisoned Planet: How to Choose Safe Food for You and Your Family* (New York: Harmony Books, 1990).
> *Perhaps the most comprehensive list of recommendations for purchasing safe food. Recommended for the truly dedicated consumer.*

Ruth Winter, M.S., *Poisons In Your Food: The Dangers You Face And What You Can Do About Them* (New York: Crown Publishers, Inc., 1969, 1991).
> *A sober discussion of food contaminants. Not for those who worry a lot.*

General Books About Food Additives

Michael F. Jacobson, Ph.D., *The Complete Eater's Digest & Nutrition Scoreboard*, Revised and Updated (Garden City, New York: Anchor Books, 1985).
> *Probably the most balanced and dependable source of information about selected additives. Also includes discussions about healthfulness and safety of different foods. Recommended.*

Ruth Winter, *A Consumer's Dictionary of Food Additives*, Newly Revised Edition (New York: Crown Publishers, Inc., 1984).
> *A exhaustive dictionary of additives, including many chemicals used in artificial flavorings. Largely critical of additives and food technology. The most thorough reference work for the general consumer.*

Books About Food and Nutrition

Boston Children's Hospital, with Susan Baker, M.D., Ph.D. and Roberta R. Henry, R.D., *Parent's Guide to Nutrition* (Reading, Massachusetts: Addison-Wesley Publishing Company, Inc., 1987).
> *A useful volume which is occasionally "establishment" oriented.*

Jane Brody, *Jane Brody's Nutrition Book*, Revised and Updated (New York: Bantam Books, 1987).
> *Informative, useful, and insistent. Subtitled: "A Lifetime Guide to Good Eating for Better Health and Weight Control by the Personal Health Columnist of **The New York Times**".*

Nikki & David Goldbeck, *The Goldbeck's Guide to Good Food* (New York: New American Library, 1987).
> *A thorough and authoritative guide for the careful consumer. Recommended.*

Earl Mindell, *Unsafe At Any Meal* (New York: Warner Books, 1987).
> *Useful but occasionally overwhelming. Hundreds of reasons to avoid eating.*

Books about Specific Topics

Anne Witte Garland, *For Our Kids' Sake: How to Protect Your Child Against Pesticides in Food* (San Francisco: Sierra Club Books, 1989)
> *A broad and informative discussion of pesticides, focussing on the needs of children. Also a manual for consumer and political action.*

(Stephanie Bernardo Johns, *The Allergy Guide to Brand-Name Foods and Food Additives* (New York: New American Library, 1988).
> *Good introduction to food allergies and allergens.*

Lawrie Mott & Karen Snyder (Natural Resources Defense Council), *Pesticide Alert: A Guide to Pesticides in Fruits and Vegetables*, (San Francisco: Sierra Club, 1987)
> *Alarming and controversial "exposé" of pesticide use in agriculture and specific agricultural products.*

John Robbins, *Diet for a New America* (Walpole, New Hampshire: Stillpoint Publishing, 1987).
> *Controversial and disturbing description of meat "production" by an heir to an ice cream fortune.*

Tony Webb, Tim Lang, and Kathleen Tucker, *Food Irradiation: Who Wants It?* (Rochester, Vermont: Thorsons Publishers, Inc., 1987).
> *Broad critique of irradiation from an international perspective. Puts irradiation in context of the modern food system.*

Selected Newsletters

University of California, Berkeley, Wellness Letter, Subscription Department, P.O. Box 420148, Palm Coast, FL 32142
> *One of the best and most balanced of the academically oriented health and medicine newsletters. A personal favorite.*

Nutrition Action Newsletter (Center for Science in the Public Interest, 1875 Connecticut Avenue, N.W., Suite 300, Washington, D.C. 20036).
> *A readable and independent health newsletter published by one of the nation's foremost consumer protection organizations.*

Organizations

Center for Science in the Public Interest, 1875 Connecticut Avenue, N.W., Suite 300, Washington, DC 20009
> *A trustworthy lobbying and consumer-information organization. Publishes a number of thoughtful resources, including* **Nutrition Action Newsletter.**

Public Voice for Food and Health Policy, 1001 Connecticut Avenue, N.W., Suite 522, Washington, DC 20036
> *A respected advocate of consumer involvement in policy-making decisions. Works effectively with government, industry, and consumers. Members receive quarterly reports and discounts on publications.*